LIFE AND EDUCATION

OF

LAURA DEWEY BRIDGMAN,

THE DEAF, DUMB, AND BLIND GIRL.

BY MARY SWIFT LAMSON.

BOSTON:

HOUGHTON, MIFFLIN AND COMPANY.

𝔗𝔥𝔢 𝔕𝔦𝔳𝔢𝔯𝔰𝔦𝔡𝔢 𝔓𝔯𝔢𝔰𝔰, 𝔆𝔞𝔪𝔟𝔯𝔦𝔡𝔤𝔢.

1890.

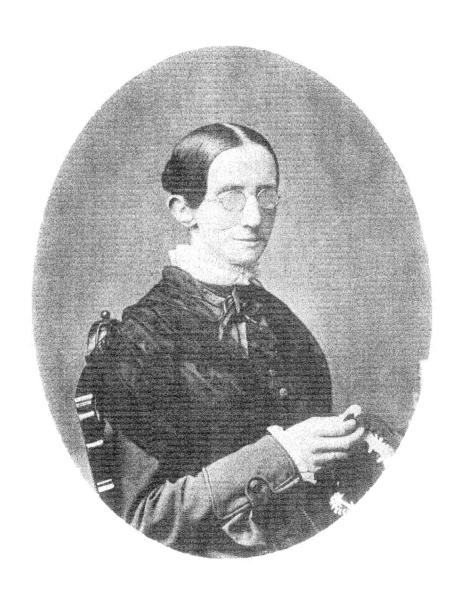

LAURA DEWEY BRIDGMAN 1878

INTRODUCTION.

THE author and editor of the present volume was a teacher for five years in the "Perkins Institution and Massachusetts Asylum for the Blind." She was for three years the special instructor of Laura Bridgman, and had the honor of giving the first lesson to Oliver Caswell, another blind and deaf mute at the Asylum. She differed from Dr. Samuel G. Howe, the director of the Asylum, in regard to the time of commencing the religious education of Laura; but she held him in high esteem as an enterprising, skilful, and persevering instuctor. He characterized her in words like the following: She is "a lady of great intelligence who is devotedly attached to" [Laura]; "an able and excellent teacher," who "fulfilled her duty with ability and conscientiousness; has been faithful and industrious; and in the intellectual instruction she has shown great tact and ability"; "indeed to Miss Swift [now Mrs. Lamson] and Miss Wight [now Mrs. Bond] belong, far more than to any other persons, the pure satisfaction of having been instrumental in the beautiful development of Laura's character." *

One noteworthy advantage has been enjoyed by the editor of this volume. She has retained an intimate acquaintance with Laura Bridgman for thirty seven years.

* Annual Reports of the Trustees of the Perkins Institution and Massachusetts Asylum for the Blind, XI, p. 37; XIII, pp. 23, 24; XIV, p. 30, etc., etc. These documents will be hereafter alluded to simply as Annual Reports.

The blind deaf-mute was only in the thirteenth year of
her age, and in the third year of her residence at the
Asylum, when she was put under the particular and
almost exclusive charge of Mrs. Lamson, and from that
day to this has been accustomed to communicate her
thoughts freely to the teacher who instructed her in
1840. The editor of the volume has thus been able to
compare the later with the earlier development of Laura.
Laura herself is liable to forget those earlier developments, to mistake her more recently acquired knowledge
for that which she had acquired at a remoter period.
The ideas, however, which she expressed in the initial
stages of her education were recorded day by day, and the
testimony of a written journal is far more trustworthy
than that of the memory.

This volume has a special value in the fact that it pre-
serves the style of the original diary; it records the progress of Laura in detail, just as the progress was, without
any attempt to embellish the history; without any attempt
to magnify the excellences or to conceal the foibles of the
blind deaf-mute; without any other generalizations than
those which were forced upon the notice of an instructor
writing for her own private use; without any theory to
defend or to impugn; without any foresight of any use
which might afterward be made of her honest record. It
would have been easy to write a sensational narrative of
so unique a person as Laura Bridgman, and to cluster
splendid panegyrics around a few salient points of her
character. To many readers such a rhapsodical style
would have been more interesting than the record of the
daily routine of her childish questions and tardy acquisi-
tions. This homely record, however, of blunders and slow
progress is more readily credited, is more valuable to the
philosopher, and more practically useful to the common
mind, than would have been the most brilliant descriptions of isolated facts in Laura's life. The wheat including

the alcohol is more wholesome than the alcohol distilled from the wheat.

The narratives of Jean Massieu leave us in an incredulous state of mind, in consequence of the fact that his marvellous exploits are recorded without a sufficiently copious detail of the processes which fitted him to perform them. Six children of his parents, three boys and three girls, were, like himself, congenital deaf-mutes. He was born in 1772 and died in 1846. At the age of thirteen years and nine months, without having exhibited any sign of eminent talents, he became a pupil of the Abbé Sicard. He doubtless acquired a great power of mind; but we are apt to overrate his genius and to receive on the whole a false impression, when we read of his bright sayings, and do not read of the dull performances intermingled with them. It seems improbable that any deaf-mute could habitually, and without distinctive preparation, give such answers as Massieu is reported to have given in some of his school exercises. We suspect that some of his answers were (like the brilliant remarks of many a modern deaf-mute) the remembered utterances of his instructors. If original, they were exceptional.

The following is one specimen of them: " What is a revolution? " [a question asked in the time of the French Reign of Terror.] " It is a tree whose roots have taken the place of its trunk." — " What is gratitude ? " " Gratitude is the memory of the heart." — " What is hope ? " " Hope is the blossom of happiness." — What is the difference between hope and desire ? " " Desire is a tree in leaf ; hope is a tree in flower ; and enjoyment is a tree in fruit." — " What is eternity ? " " A day without yesterday or to-morrow; a line that has no ends." — " What is time ? " " A line that has two ends ; a path which begins in the cradle and ends in the tomb." — " What is God ? " " The necessary being, the sun of eternity, the mechanist of nature, the eye of justice, the watchmaker of the universe, the soul of the world." — " Does God reason ? " [a question proposed to Massieu by Sir James Mackintosh.] " Man reasons because he doubts ; he deliberates, he decides. God is omniscient ; he knows all things ; he never doubts ; he therefore never reasons."

We do not claim that Laura Bridgman has a genius equal to that of Massieu ; but we do not deem it impossible to cull out from her conversation, as recorded in the present volume, such remarks as would keep the reader in a state of constant surprise at her sagacity. These isolated remarks would attract more admiration but would yield less instruction than they do now. A few specimens of fruits, at a horticultural fair, may make an entirely erroneous impression in regard to the substantial produce of the garden.

The earliest notice which I have seen of Laura Bridgman is from the pen of that excellent and eminent man, Dr. Reuben Dimond Mussey, Professor of Anatomy and Surgery at Dartmouth College. His letter is important because it was written six months before the blind deaf-mute entered the asylum at Boston, and because it gives suggestive information in regard to her natural capabilities and her early moral developments. As the first home of Laura was at Hanover, N. H., the seat of Dartmouth College, the character of herself and family could be easily learned by Prof. Mussey, and so careful an observer as he would not have placed undue reliance on their testimony. The letter * was written in reply to one received from a distinguished instructor of the deaf and dumb, and is as follows : —

HANOVER. N. H., April 14, 1837.

Dear Sir: The blind and deaf child, referred to in your letter received this morning, is, I presume, the same who

---

* It was published in the Twenty-first Report of the American Asylum, at Hartford, etc., pp. 41, 42.

lives within this township, seven miles from our village. I have ridden out to-day and passed an hour at her father's, and have obtained from her parents the following particulars: —

Her name is Laura D. Bridgman; seven years old; a girl of middling stature for her age, and of a pretty uniform health. When about two years old she lost her hearing altogether, and all distinctness of vision, by scarlet fever. She has never [since] given evidence of hearing any sort of sound, but she can perceive light enough to enable her to tell where the windows are during the day, and is attracted by a lighted taper at evening. A white cloth or a sheet of white paper, placed near to her right eye so as to reflect a strong light, engages her attention; so does the hand, waved from side to side between her eye and the window. The left eye is wholly destroyed. A scarlet colored cloth put into her hand seemed to make a slight impression, as if she received the feeblest notion of color from it. After she was somewhat fatigued, however, I placed a sheet of white paper before her eye and moved it from side to side several times, evidently without her being conscious of it. She has, probably, no reminiscence of sounds or of visual objects from impressions received before the attack of scarlet fever. She was considered by her parents as unusually intelligent before her sickness, and is still so regarded by them. Specimens of her knitting and sewing were shown me which looked very well. Much of her time is employed in knitting; indeed, she is uneasy when out of employment, and if allowed would attempt to do most kinds of work in the house which she finds others doing. She sets the dinner-table, laying the plates and knives and forks in their places and in number corresponding with the number of the family. The particular plate and knife and fork used by her little brother she is sure to put in the right place.

Her fondness for dress is as remarkable as that of any

child that can see. New clothes give her great pleasure. She knows every article of dress belonging to her mother, and is gratified when her mother puts on her best dresses. She is as fond of society as of dress, and is most untiring in her exercises with her playmates.

A silver pencil-case, for the first time, was handed her to-day, while I was present. She very soon learned to unscrew and replace the head-piece, and the part containing the lead. This was a new thing, which clearly gave her great pleasure, as she occasionally smiled, and had her whole attention absorbed with it for some time.

She is kind and affectionate in her disposition ; with her two brothers younger than she, the only children of the family besides herself, she is always ready to divide fruit or any other pleasant eatable which is presented to her. Her resentments are keen, but transitory, and her parents can easily persuade her by patting her head to submit to their direction. Her mother says that in this way the child can be induced to take the most disgusting medicines, as rhubarb, tincture of aloes, etc.

Her sense of smell is thought by her mother to be less acute than that of other children, as she very seldom applies an odorous substance to her nose ; it is not improbable that this sense may have been impaired by the fever. The senses of taste and of touch, which last is very acute, appear to be the only inlets of knowledge, with the exception of the extremely dim vision before mentioned, which is too imperfect to enable her to avoid objects even in a strong light.

Very sincerely yours,

R. D. MUSSEY.

This letter of Professor Mussey is more significant than it may appear to be at first sight. When he speaks of the sense of touch (which was, in fact, Laura's main organ for communication with the material world), he doubtless

Includes not merely the " touch proper," but also the capacity for the " acute " sensations, pleasant or painful ; also for the sensations of pressure and weight, of temperature ; also for the " muscular sensations," those of the rough, smooth, slippery, adhesive, elastic, non-elastic, etc. ; all those sensations which are commonly assigned to the touch in its general and loose meaning. From the Professor's suggestive letter it appears that Laura Bridgman retained her power of vision, hearing, taste, and smell until she was " about [in actual fact she was a little more than] two years old "; that she retained a power of indistinct vision until she was over seven years old; that her parents had noticed her deficiency in the sense of smell, but had not noticed her deficiency in the sense of taste, after she had become a deaf-mute. She was easily persuaded to take " the most disgusting medicines." Dr. Mussey does not appear to have suspected the cause. When she came to the Boston Asylum she was unable, at least occasionally, to distinguish rhubarb from tea by the taste. Still, the power of this sense, as that of smell, seems to have been somewhat variable. In her fifteenth year she could, at certain times, distinguish certain articles of food by smelling them. At particular periods she detected the fragrance of a flower. When we read, as we sometimes do, that " from her tenderest infancy she could neither smell, taste, hear, nor see," we must qualify the remark ; it is convenient but not strictly accurate ; it must be explained to mean that soon after she entered on her third year she lost entirely her sense of hearing (therefore her power of speaking), and in large measure her sense of taste and that of smell ; that after the beginning of her eighth year she lost entirely her sense of sight, and this had been so indistinct as to be comparatively useless after the beginning of her third year.

In several particulars, then, her case is unique. It is not very uncommon for deaf-mutes to have an impaired

sense of taste and also of smell. Both of these senses are
so connected with the sense of hearing that the same
cause which disorders the latter may disorder also the two
former.   Often the Swiss crétin is not only unable to
speak and to hear, but is also unable to taste and to smell
as accurately or as keenly as other persons. The crétin.
however, is deficient in intellect, as Laura Bridgman is
not.

The loss of vision alone is not generally attended with
an impaired sense of taste, and is often attended with an
unusual keenness in the sense of smell. Perhaps there
has never been another instance than this of Laura Bridgman in which the loss of sight has been combined with
the entire loss of hearing and also with a loss of two other
senses. Probably there have been more instances than
are recorded in which the loss of sight has been combined
with deafness and dumbness. Perhaps the great majority
of blind deaf-mutes have been destroyed by the neglect
or the violence of their relatives. In ancient legal treat-
ises they are recognized as idiots. Dr. Howe quotes *
from Blackstone's Commentaries the following passage :
" A man is not an idiot, if he hath any glimmerings of
reason so that he can tell his parents, his age, or the like
matters. But a man who is born deaf, dumb, and blind is
looked upon by the law as in the same state with an idiot :
he being supposed incapable of any understanding, as
wanting all those senses which furnish the human mind
with ideas."

Modern history has given us a more or less particular
account of at least fifteen persons who have lived deaf,
dumb, and blind. It is rather remarkable that the cele.
brated Abbé de l'Epée had never heard of one such person. Still, supposing it possible that individuals should
be born unable either to see or to hear, he contrived a

---

* In Annual Report, IX, pp. 34, 35.

process of educating them. The process, although described more than a hundred years ago, reminds us of the
method in which Laura Bridgman was instructed. The
blind deaf-mute was to have an alphabet of polished steel ·
the letters composing the name of some sensible object
were to be felt by the fingers of one hand, while the object
itself was to be felt by the fingers of the other. The il-
lustrious M. Sicard, who was the successor of the Abbé de
l'Epée in the office of instructing the deaf and dumb, proposed that if the blind deaf-mute were desirous of obtaining any particular article, it should be withheld from him
until he had spelled the name of it. He should not taste
the peach or the plum until he had arranged the letters
composing those words. The blind deaf-mutes in the
Boston Asylum were occasionally stimulated by the same
appeals to their appetite. In this way Laura Bridgman
would sometimes attempt to instruct some other pupil
who could neither see nor hear the name of the desired
edible. She demanded the letters of the word *c a k e* before she would give the cake to the blind and deaf learner.
It is substantially an old custom, pursued by parents with
their children and by children with each other. Indeed,
there have been "select schools," where the scholars were
taught their letters by the use of a gingerbread alphabet,
which was to be devoured as soon as its literary significance had been thoroughly digested. We strangely forget
that the deaf-mutes and the blind deaf-mutes are human
beings and are to be treated as other human beings; they
are influenced by the same motives which affect the race
in general, and are to be educated on the same principles
which regulate the education of ordinary scholars. The
special difficulty is in opening an avenue to their minds.
When we have once penetrated the wall which has separated them from us, there is no more *real* mystery in teaching them than in teaching other persons. There is a mystery in the mental progress of *every* child : in the menta.

progress of the blind deaf-mute the mystery is greater in *degree* and is longer continued ; but in *kind* it is the same mystery.   To succeed in the first step is the peculiar difficulty.   " Principium dimidium facti."

The narrative of Laura Bridgman reminds us that all art, as well as all science, has been progressive.   Aristotle borrowed much from his now forgotten predecessors. Kepler opened the door for Newton.   No art springs complete from the brain of any man.   The present methods of instructing the blind were not first suggested by the Abbé Haüy in the last century, but the principle which regulates them had long before his day been familiar to the mind of educators.   Narratives almost fabulous had been given of blind men feeling and thus reading the words of a book or manuscript.   So the present methods of instructing the deaf and dumb were not invented between 1712 and 1789, by the Abbé de l'Epée, without any hint from a previous writer.   They were suggested to him by a Spanish treatise which was written in 1590, and was thrown in his way by accident.   Indeed, as early as 1485, Rodolphus Agricola, describing " the immense and almost incredible power of the human mind," instances as little less than miraculous what he himself had witnessed, — a person deaf from infancy, and consequently dumb, who had learned to understand writing. and, as if possessed of speech, was able to write down his whole thoughts.   The first art of instructing the blind in letters, and the second art of instructing the deaf-mute, are compounded with each other in the art of instructing those who are both blind and also deaf and dumb.   The principle regulating this combination was ingeniously stated by George Dalgarno (sometimes written Dalgarus), a Scotchman, who wrote in 1680 on the education of deaf-mutes, and from whom more than one renowned scholar has borrowed more than he has acknowledged.   His suggestive words are, ' The soul can exert her powers by the ministry of any of the senses; and, therefore, when she is deprived of her principal secretaries, the eye and the ear, then she must be contented with the service of her lackeys and scullions, the other senses, which are no less true and faithful to their mistress than the eye and the ear, but not so quick for despatch. . . . And as 1 think the eye to be as docile as the ear, so neither see I any reason but the hand might be made as tractable an organ as the tongue, and as soon brought to form, if not fair, at least legible characters, as the tongue to imitate and echo back articulate sounds." * Notwithstanding his expressed confidence, it would have surprised this learned Scotchman to be told that two centuries after he penned the sentences above quoted, there would be living in the New World a woman who had lost four " secretaries " of the mind, and yet, mainly by means of the tips of her fingers, her only remaining " lackeys " and " scullions," she could express ideas as rapidly as an ordinary penman could record them.

Prof. Mussey, in his letter respecting Laura Bridgman, speaks of the practical skill which she had acquired before she was educated at the Asylum. Other instances of like skill are readily suggested to us. In Dugald Stewart's account of the so-called blind deaf-mute, James Mitchell, we read, " He had received a severe wound in his foot, and during its cure he usually sat by the fireside with his foot resting on a small footstool. More than a year afterwards, a servant boy, with whom he used to play, was obliged to confine himself to a chair from a similar cause. Young Mitchell, perceiving that his companion remained longer in one situation than he used to do, examined him attentively, and seemed quickly to discover, by the band-

---

* Works of Dugald Stewart, Vol. III, p. 325, Ed. 1829; Edinburgh Review, Vol LXI, pp. 407, 417.

ages on his foot, the reason of his confinement. Hé immediately walked up stairs to a garret, sought out, amidst
several other pieces of furniture, the little footstool which
had formerly supported his own wounded limb, and gently
placed the servant-boy's foot upon it." *　James Mitchell
had been educated by the use of natural signs to perform
such exploits.

Thomas Whipple, M.D., a physician in Wentworth, New
Hampshire, in a letter dated Feb. 28, 1834, has given the
following account of Samuel Elbridge Eames, who became
deaf, dumb, and blind when he was about two years old,
and died when he was sixteen years six months and
twenty-three days old : " His father missed an axe, and
had [missed it] for some time; not being able to find it, he
suspected the boy had hidden it. His mother made him
feel another axe, and patted him, and made some motions
with him ; he went into an unfinished part of the house,
took up a loose floor-board, and brought forward the axe.
He went into his father's gig-wagon on a certain time and
took all the ruffs from the screws which held the parts of
the wagon together ; on being discovered he began and
replaced them, not misplacing a single one He has taken
a bunch of keys consisting of six, and opened his father's
desk, and would do it as readily as any one of the family. . .
I visited his father, who was sick. He detected my manner
of opening and shutting the door by the jar which he felt;
he met me, felt me over from head to foot, smelt my clothes
and saddle-bags, followed me into the sick-room, took my
saddle-bags on my putting them down, opened them, raised
the vial-case, opened it, took out one of the vials, uncorked
it, smelt of its contents, shook his head, and would not
taste ; then replaced the vial and returned everything to
its first state. After this trial, though nothing was done
to deter him, he would not on my visiting at the house

---

* Works of Dugald Stewart, Vol. III, p. 309, Amer. Ed. 1829.

open the saddle-bags, but would, on smelling them, leave them." *

It would have been impossible for a blind deaf-mute to perform works like these had he not been previously educated by means of natural signs. We are thus reminded of the fact that all processes of instruction depend ultimately on natural language. This is the basis on which arbitrary language is founded. Men must have some means of communication before they learn the use of spoken or written words. They have an instinctive tendency to perform outward actions, and to express their thoughts and feelings by smiles, frowns, or other movements of the body. They detect the resemblance between their own expressions and the expressions of other persons. So they learn the thoughts and feelings of other persons. Some of these expressions are probably understood by intuition and without a reasoning process. Mr. Coleridge says, "There is in the heart of all men a working principle, call it ambition, or vanity, or desire of distinction, the inseparable adjunct of our individuality and personal nature, and flowing from the same source as language, the instinct and necessity in each man of declaring his particular existence, and thus of singularizing himself." If he cannot do this by conventional words he will do it by instinctive signs. We must not suppose, however, that the use of conventional words is less really the ordinance of God than is the use of instinctive signs. He has made us not only with the power, but also with the decisive tendencies to use articulate speech. We are inclined by a law of nature (and this in the last resort is God) to express thought by words as its symbols. What we call natural language is his direct gift ; what we call artificial language is his indirect gift. As a man is im·

---

* Twenty-first Report of the Directors of the American Asylum at Hartford, pp. 35, 36.

pelled to put forth a choice of this or that, but he has a power of putting forth a choice of either rather than the other, in a similar way man is impelled to use this or that artificial sign of his ideas, but he may use one or a different one as it pleases him. The Book of Genesis was not designed to teach philology; but the nineteenth verse of the second chapter intimates that Adam had an impulse to name the animals around him, and the particular designation of each animal was left to his free choice. Although a person be unable to speak, or to hear a word if he should speak it, or to see a movement of the vocal organs of other men, yet he has an impulse, whenever he is excited, to use his own vocal organs; not only to use them for the sake of relieving a pressure on the lungs, or giving to the larynx such an exercise as its health or comfort requires, but for the sake of marking the distinction between one object and another. He has an impulse to emit vocal sounds distinct from the unintelligible screams, groans, yells, of many deaf-mutes. " Natural language is the servant of the heart; [arbitrary] speech is the handmaid of the intellect." The history of Laura Bridgman illustrates these principles. " So strong seems the tendency to utter vocal sounds that Laura uses them for different persons of her acquaintance whom she meets, having a distinct sound for each one. When after a short absence she goes into the sitting-room where there are a dozen blind girls, she embraces them by turn, uttering rapidly and in a high key the peculiar sound which designates each one ; and so different are they (the sounds uttered by her) that any of the blind girls can tell whom she is with." * Dr. Lieber says, " Laura has near sixty sounds for persons. When her teacher asked her, at my suggestion, how many sounds she recollected, she produced at once twenty-seven. Three of her

---

* Tenth Annual Report, p. 32.

teachers, Dr. Howe included, stated to me that she had certainly from fifty to sixty." * The impulse to utter a sound as the distinctive name of her friend seemed to come first; the translation of it into her finger language came second. After having employed one sound ("noise") for the lady when unmarried, she saw the propriety of employing a different sound ("noise") for the same lady when married. She was not encouraged at the Asylum to use what is called the natural nor the analogical language; her thoughts, which might have flowed out in some kind of pantomime, were directed by her teachers into the channel of the arbitrary language of the fingers; and through this channel they flowed easily and rapidly. "She often talks with herself, *sometimes holding long conversations, speaking with one hand and replying with the other.*" † After all, the impulse to utter audible words could not be repressed. Not only the comfort of the mind, but the health of the body is promoted by yielding to this impulse. The instincts of man correspond with his power of thought and with his animal structure; and all are the contrivance of the Mind which intended that man should be an articulately speaking, as well as an articulately thinking, animal.

The history of Laura Bridgman casts some light on the doctrine of intuitions. We must here confine ourselves to the inquiry whether, before her instruction at the Asylum, she had an idea of and a belief in the infinite God and her own immortality. Throughout his Reports, Dr. Howe has expressed the confident opinion that she had no idea of the Infinite Being, of course no belief in him. This opinion seems to be correct. Fifteen years ago I

---

* A Paper on the Vocal Sounds of Laura Bridgman, p. 26. By Francis Lieber. Smithsonian Contributions, etc.

† A Paper on the Vocal Sounds of Laura Bridgman, p. 30. By Francis Lieber. Smithsonian Contributions, etc.

had two interviews (one of them much prolonged) with her in regard to her notions of the Supreme Being. It appeared evident, first, that before she entered the Asylum she had no belief in the existence of an infinite and perfect Deity, and no idea of him ; secondly, that her habit (an uncommonly obvious one) of reasoning from effect to cause, and from the phenomena of her own moral nature, led her to believe, occasionally, in some mysterious being or beings by whom her interests were affected ; thirdly, that her idea of this being or these beings was far inferior to an idea of the infinite God, and was just as lofty or just as low, as her observation of phenomena had been exact and extensive or loose and limited ; fourthly, that as her belief depended upon and resulted from her observation of phenomena, it would have risen to a belief in the infinite One if she had taken a comprehensive and an accurate view of these phenomena. Whatever faith she had was not intuitive in the ordinary sense of that word, but came from reasoning ; this faith fell below a belief in the true God, because the data for reasoning had been imperfectly examined. Still, in the above-mentioned interviews, it was apparent that her sensibilities had been unsatisfied in consequence of her want of religious knowledge, and that as soon as this want was supplied at the Asylum the demands of her constitution were happily met. In this particular there was an instructive difference between Laura Bridgman and Julia Brace, the blind deaf-mute of the Hartford Asylum. "The following experiment has lately been tried [on Julia Brace, when she was about twenty years of age] : Her attention was called to a great variety of artificial objects, and she was told that Miss C. made this, Mr. S. that ; a man one, a woman another, and so on. The idea of making is familiar, for she makes some things herself. Then, a number of natural objects were presented her, such as minerals, fruits, flowers, plants, vegetables, and she was told that neither this friend nor that acquaintance made any of them ; that neither men nor women made them. The hope was entertained that her curiosity would be excited, and that a way might be discovered to convey to her mind the great idea of the Almighty Creator. The attempt was not successful, and though several times repeated, has not as yet resulted in exciting her mind, fixing her attention, or giving us any encouraging indications." * Even at this late day, when Julia Brace is more than seventy years old, it is difficult to determine how far her mind has advanced in apprehending the true character of God. If she had been as ready as Laura to infer an ordinary cause from an ordinary event, she might have been as ready as Laura to appreciate what was told her in regard to the infinite and ultimate Cause of all events.

As Miss Bridgman had no intuitive idea of the Supreme Being, so she had none of the soul's immortality. In the interviews referred to above, I could not find that, before her instruction at the Asylum, she had any proper idea of death. She described, with almost frantic gestures, the horror which she felt when, before she was seven years old, she touched a corpse ; but the horror arose not from a just notion of the *corpse*, but from her new sensations of the coldness and unbending stiffness of the body. As she did not think of death, so she did not think of existence *after* death. Without an idea of mortality, she was without any proper idea of immortality. As she had never thought of an infinite mind, so she had never thought of an eternal duration. Of course she expected to exist from day to day, as she expected that the earth would continue from day to day. If we regard her expectation of living in the future as an expectation of immortal life, then we must regard her expectation of the earth's contin-

* Twenty-first Report of the Directors of the Hartford Asylum, 1837, p. 28.

uance in the future as an expectation of its continuance forever. We have, moreover, as much right to say that she had an *intuitive* belief in the continued existence of her parents' farm-house as to say that she had an *intuitive* belief in the continued existence of her own soul. Indeed, I could not learn that, before she was instructed at the Asylum, she had formed any idea of the soul as distinct from the body. Even at the Asylum her *first* apprehension of the spirit, as different from bone and muscle, appeared to be an apprehension of the breath which, at the mortal hour, was taken by the great Spirit from the body.

The history of Laura Bridgman illustrates the importance of a symmetrical development of the human powers and sensibilities. It is not uncommon to hear men say that John Milton was indebted to his blindness for his fame ; that Sanderson, Moyes, and Huber would have accomplished less than they have, if they had not been deprived of vision. It is said of the noted Puritan, Dr. John Guyse, that he "lost his eyesight in the pulpit while he was at prayer before the sermon, but nevertheless managed to preach as usual." He was told by one of his hearers, " God be praised that your sight is gone ! I never heard [you] preach so powerful a [sermon] in my life. I wish for my own part that the Lord had taken away your sight twenty years ago ; for your ministry would have been more useful by twenty degrees." " Malebranche, when he wished to think intensely, used to close his windows-shutters in the daytime, excluding every ray of light ; and for a like reason Democritus is said to have put out his eyes, in order that he might philosophize the better, — which latter story, however, it should be observed, .hough told by several ancient writers, is doubted by Cicero and discredited by Plutarch." *

---

* Edinburgh Review, Vol. XCIX, p. 62.

It is doubtless true that the deprivation of sight and hearing will occasionally stimulate the mind to augmented exertion in order to overcome the disadvantage. This fact proves that the deprivation *is* a disadvantage. It is also true that blindness and deafness free the soul from many distractions; but the evil of these distractions is incomparably less than the evil of exclusion from the exhilarating influence of sight and sound. Destitute of the spiritualizing, refining influences exerted by the eye and ear, the blind deaf-mute is tempted to an excessive indulgence of his lower animal nature. He is apt to be embittered by a sense of his privations, for his endowments are as far inferior to those of the mere deaf-mute as the endowments of the deaf-mute are inferior to those of the hearer and speaker. He is also prone to be irritated by the toil which he must undergo in learning what others learn with ease. If we try the experiment of attempting to find our way around the walls of a room completely dark, when we did not know exactly from what part of the room we started, we are surprised at our inability to learn our bearings, to judge of the relations between the walls, chairs, and doors, with which one glance of the eye would make us perfectly familiar. The blind deaf-mute is subjected to the same kind, but a greater degree of irritation in attempting to *orienteer* himself in any department of knowledge. Then the monotony of his labors is annoying If Laura Bridgman had been able to see and hear, to smell and taste, as others do, she might have been often diverted from her studies by processions of soldiers, by the music of birds, by the fragrance of flowers, and the flavor of fruits. Free from these distractions, her mind could be almost as intent on her arithmetic by night as by day, in her walks as at her fireside, in a conservatory of roses and at a luxurious dinner-table as in her school. The whole world was to her a continuous school. But this monotony of mental action brought multiplied annoyances. Equal annoyances came from the necessity of her dependence upon herself. Many of her shades of doubt could not be indicated *by* her, and many shades of the wisdom, gathered in the books, could not be expressed *to* her. Her mind was like a child led without a lantern by a tenuous thread through the catacombs, the thread often broken, the leader often lost. We are apt to fail of appreciating the emphasis of such words as were often impressed by her fingers on the fingers of her teacher. These words were a real *wail* for clearer thoughts; they were loud *cries* for the removal of her mental perplexities. Sir James Mackintosh speaks of the pain which James Mitchell was liable to suffer " from the occasional violences of a temper irritated by a fruitless struggle to give utterance to his thoughts and wishes, disturbed still further by the vehemence of those gestures which he employs to supply the deficiency of his signs, and released from that restraint on anger which we experience when we see and hear its excesses disapproved by our fellow-creatures."* Similar remarks are applicable to Laura Bridgman, who has been doomed to ever-recurring disappointments.

Some may suppose that her deficiency in the senses of smell and taste was no disadvantage to her intellect; but the want of any physical sense is such a disadvantage, other things being equal. The mind is delicately poised among a variety of physical powers, and any disarrangement of any one of these powers disturbs the mental activity. Many a fresh train of thought has been started by the odors of a garden, by the taste of its fruit. The mind and heart have been quickened by the incense at a Catholic altar, and by the flavor of the viands at a religious festival. " I am mortified," said an eminent scholar, " when I reflect on the influence of one peach in refreshing my mind for study. Some of the most significant words relating to the human mind (the word *sagacity*, for instance) are

---

* **Works of Dugald Stewart, Vol. III, Ed. 1829, p. 345.**

borrowed from this very sense [of smell], and the conspic-
uous place which its sensations occupy in the poetical
language of all nations shows how easily and naturally
they ally themselves with the refined operations of the
fancy and the moral emotions of the heart. The infinite
variety of modifications, besides, of which they are suscep-
tible, might furnish useful resources, in the way of asso-
ciation for prompting the memory, where it stood in need
of assistance. One of the best schools for the education
of such a pupil (a blind deaf-mute) would probably be a
well-arranged botanic garden." *

It is obvious that in certain particulars Laura Bridgman suffered many disadvantages in comparison with
those which have fallen to the lot of other blind deaf-
mutes. Thus James Mitchell was not entirely blind nor
entirely deaf, and his two kindred senses of smell and taste
were remarkably acute. Once, when his sister's shoes were
wet, he first perceived the fact by his sense of smell, then
felt them, and insisted on her changing them. When any
new object was put into his hands he first examined it
with the tips of his fingers, and then insinuated " his
tongue into all its inequalities, thus using it [the tongue]
an an organ of touch as well as taste." †

It is common to compare Laura Bridgman with Julia
Brace. This woman was born June 13, 1807; was ad-
mitted to the Hartford Asylum when she was eighteen
years of age. She became entirely deaf and blind at the
age of four years and about five months. At that time
she could read and spell words of two syllables. Her
sense of smell, like that of many other blind persons, is
wonderfully acute. She has been frequently known to
select her own clothes from a mass of dresses belonging to a hundred and thirty or forty persons. " Her

---

* Dugald Stewart's Works, Vol. III, p. 315, Ed. 1829.
† Dugald Stewart's Works, Vol. III, p. 337, Ed. 1829.

manner is to examine each article by feeling; but to decide upon it by the sense of smell, and in regard to her
own things she never errs." * She has been frequently
known to discriminate, merely by smelling them, the
recently washed stockings of the boys from those of the
girls at the Asylum. Among a hundred and twenty or
thirty teaspoons used at the Asylum she could distinguish those of the steward from those of the pupils,
"though a casual observer would hardly notice the difference.† It has been stated that by putting the eye of a
cambric needle upon the tip of her tongue, she could feel
the thread as it entered the eye and pressed upon her
tongue, and she would thus thread the needle. These instances prove that her sense of touch was at least equal,
while that of smell was far superior, to those of Laura
Bridgman. It must not be forgotten, however, that in
certain particulars Laura Bridgman enjoyed advantages
superior to these of some other blind deaf-mutes. During
the first two years of her life her physical senses and powers
were equal to those of other children; in her eighth year
she would detect a very bright color. Although James
Mitchell had through life a faint sensation of sight and
also of hearing, yet he was born almost blind and deaf;
others have been born entirely so. A person who has once
had the sensations of flavor and fragrance, light and sound,
is not exactly the same person he would have been without
these sensations. They must have given some impulse to
his mind; they must have started him in his progress of
thought. Laura Bridgman was born in lowly life, but
was early surrounded with better influences than those
which were exerted on some whose avenues of knowledge
were blocked up like hers. More than seven years of her

---

* Twenty-first Report of the Directors of the Hartford Asylum
p. 24.

† Twenty-first Report of the Hartford Asylum, p. 23.

early childhood were spent in the vicinity of Dartmouth College. She probably received no direct influence from the college, still the atmosphere of a New England town, in which a literary institution like Dartmouth has existed for a century, is more healthful to the soul than the atmosphere of the almshouses in which several of the blind deaf-mutes have been condemned to live. Before she was eight years old she was placed under the general superintendence of Dr. Samuel G. Howe, and during twelve subsequent years she was under the care of some accomplished instructor, specially and almost exclusively devoted to this one pupil. She had a particular trait distinguishing her above the great majority of all those with whom it can be of any use to compare her. This trait was an uncommon love of knowledge. Inquisitiveness makes the scholar. A difference in the degree of curiosity causes an incalculable difference in the degree of mental improvement, between one pupil and another.

If her curiosity had been earlier gratified in receiving a knowledge of God, her mind would have been more rapidly as well as more symmetrically developed. If the sense of smell or taste has an intellectual use, much more has the principle of religiosity.

The history of Laura Bridgman suggests a lesson on the importance of early education. We have read of a student who inquired, "Is it of any use to know Latin?" The answer was, "It is of great use to have forgotten Latin." It is very evident that Laura Bridgman forgot a large part of the education which she received before she went to the Asylum. What lasting benefit could she have derived from her first *two* years, when she saw, heard, smelled, tasted, as well as other children; from her first *seven* years, when she had some faint sensation of color, as well as of flavor and fragrance? Much advantage. An education, even if afterward forgotten, is a singular boon.

At first the infant sees everything double, everything upside down, everything in close contact with his eye. It is by a process of comparing the sensations of touch with those of sight that he learns the real position and distance and number of the objects which he sees. He listens to the song of a bird, and at length judges of its direction and remoteness from him by comparing his first sensations of touch and sight with those of hearing. He becomes familiar with these various processes of judgment and reasoning long before he is capable of analyzing them, or of retaining them for any length of time in definite remembrance. During the first two or three years of his life, he acquires a larger number of ideas, in regard to space, time, form, substance. quality, matter, mind, language, than he will acquire during any two or three years subsequent. If the child could make known his mental processes as they are performed day by day during the first five years of his life, he would be the instructor of the wisest psychologist ; he would settle the questions of the schools in regard to our original ideas, intuitions, processes of abstracting, generalizing, etc   We have read of persons solving intricate mathematical problems or explaining obscure metaphysical theories at the age of four years. We are astonished at their precocity: we should be more astonished if we should know all the moral reflections of children who are not precocious, and who are not old enough to express their thoughts in worthy language The profoundest meditations of a man, much more of a small boy, are often concealed because they do not suggest adequate words. As the scientific discoveries of little children, so have their moral reflections a life-long influence. In regard to moral truths, " What is learned in the cradle lasts to the grave." Hence. Virgil says, "*Adeo in teneris consuescere multum est.*" In one of his papers contributed to the Society for the Diffusion of Useful Knowledge, Lord Brougham pronounces his opinion that a child before his fifth year has already formed that character which it is difficult, if not morally impossible, to change. If a child's character be confirmed thus early, his education must begin earlier still. It must begin before he can understand the influences which are exerted upon him. As he cannot remember the hour when he began to distinguish a superficies from a solid, so he cannot remember the hour when he began to approve the right and to disapprove the wrong. But at that early hour he was beginning to form a habit which, like every other habit, has a tendency to be permanent. Hence the great multitude of the proverbs in various languages: "Bend the willow while it is young"; "As the twig, so the tree," etc., etc. "Education," says a writer in "Fraser's Magazine," "does not commence with the alphabet; it begins with a mother's look, with a father's smile of approbation or sign of reproof, with a sister's gentle pressure of the hand or a brother's noble act of forbearance, with birds' nests admired and not touched, with creeping ants and almost impossible emmets, with humming bees and great bee-hives, with pleasant walks and shady lanes, and with thoughts directed in sweet and kindly tones and words to mature acts of benevolence, to deeds of virtue, and to the source of all good, — to God himself."

The history of Laura Bridgman gives us new suggestions on the worth of human nature. The more clearly we see the power of the soul, so much the more keenly do we feel the need of educating it. The results which have come from the training of this disabled woman foreshadow the results which might ensue if equal labor were expended in the training of persons who are free from her disabilities. The success of her teachers is a stimulus and encouragement to all who find obstacles in imparting knowledge to others. Dr. Howe defined obstacles as " things to be overcome."

In order to estimate properly the greatness of Nature's work, it is advisable now and then to reduce the scale of them in our imagination. We cannot easily appreciate the magnitude of our earth, with its diameter of seven thousand nine hundred and twenty-five miles; of Uranus, with its diameter of thirty-five thousand miles ; of Saturn, with its diameter of seventy-six thousand and sixty-eight miles; of Jupiter, with its diameter of eighty-seven thousand miles. We must humble our views in order to exalt them. We can form a more vivid idea of the solar system, if we ever and anon imagine the earth to be but one mile in diameter, and the other planets to be proportionally small, than if we always attempt to form such images of the globes as shall accord with their actual size. When we reduce the earth to a half-inch in diameter, and reduce the other planets, the satellites, and the sun to a proportionate littleness, we prepare ourselves to form a still more exact·idea of the greatness of those orbs. Hence, the use of the planetarium. Sir John Herschell says, " As to getting correct notions on [the magnitudes and distances of the planets] by drawing circles on paper. or, still worse, from those very childish toys called orreries, it is out of the question." As to getting *perfect* notions on any great subject in this world. it is out of the question ; but *right* ideas are often suggested where they are not expressed. If we bend low, we may afterward rise high. It is said of Pope Sixtus V that while a cardinal. he walked like an old man, with his head inclined toward the ground, but as soon as he had obtained the papal tiara, which had been the object of his ambition, he assumed an erect stature and walked with a firm step. To the question, " Why this change ? " his reported answer was, " While I was looking for the keys of St. Peter, I needed to stoop; but now that I have found them, I may stand upright." We need to stoop low in order to detect the sublimity of the human soul.

When we see a girl in lowly life, "a silent, helpless, hopeless unit of mortality," whose faculties lay slumbering in a prison barred by four thick walls, not a ray of the sun's light entering her dungeon after she was eight or nine years old, not a sound of a human voice penetrating it, with but few odors wafted into it from the flowers of the field, with only a faint and feeble sense of the most luscious fruits; a lonely girl, doomed to form her notions of the outer world by what is commonly called the sense of touch, wisdom at all other entrances being almost, although not "quite shut out," who yet learns to perform operations far surpassing those of such men as can see and hear and smell and taste, we are surprised at the reserved forces belonging to human nature and exceeding some of the capabilities which are developed in common life.

In the narrative of this remarkable person, we are told of her physical exploits, which are certainly equal to those performed by James Mitchell or Samuel Eames or Julia Brace; and of her mental and moral advancement, which, in a soul so firmly imprisoned, is altogether unprecedented. She can read words which we cannot. She can detect the emphasis of a bodily motion which gives no idea to us. In the darkness of midnight she can peruse her Bible. If she were amid the roar of a battle-field, she could pursue her studies undisturbed. She *feels* a command in one movement of the arm, a permission in another movement, a reproof in a different one; an expression of impatience in one muscle, of anger in another, of esteem in a different one. She can *touch* the smiles of a congregation. She can feel the beaming of the eyes of her visitors. She can distinguish the various *tones* of various movements of the fingers. If her quick discernment of muscular expression were combined with the common powers of vision, hearing, and speech, she would be distinguished above her race as an observer of its mental phenomena. We read of men who having eyes see not, and having ears hear not; but we now behold a woman who has no eyes, and yet sees the finger of nature pointing to its God; has no ears, and yet listens to the tones of nature expressing the majesty of God; lives in the land of silence and the land of darkness, is unable to utter the name of Him who dwelleth only in the light, and yet she holds and enjoys communion with that Infinite Intelligence. The most disabled of men is made but little lower than the angels.

EDWARDS A. PARK,
Andover Theological Seminary.

AUGUST 5, 1878

PREFACE.

In a paper on the vocal sounds of Laura Bridgman, published thirty years ago, Dr. Francis Lieber expressed the hope that a general account of her education would not much longer be withheld from the public. Dr. Howe has often intimated in conversation, as well as in his annual reports, his intention to prepare such an account, but his life closed before it was accomplished. Soon after his death applications were made to the writer from various parts of the country to take up the work at once, lest that which was considered to be of much importance to the scholar be lost irretrievably.

Most reluctantly have I yielded to these requests, appreciating fully my own inability to fill the place which rightfully belonged to him who first devised a way to pour light into a mind thus darkened. My aim will be simply to state facts, and in making selections from the daily reports of her teachers to omit nothing which can be of service in any department of science. Believing that the value of the work is to be measured by its accuracy, I have carefully ascertained all dates, and have secured from most reliable sources a full account of her early teaching.

I have quoted largely from the reports of Dr. Howe (now nearly out of print), which contain a summary of her progress from year to year, and thus have preserved them from utter loss, while adding greatly to the interest of these notes.

To others is left the work of gleaning from these fruit-ful fields. There are rich sheaves for the teacher who makes the subject of language a study, and for the men tal and moral philosopher, who will find much that is val-uable each in his own department; while all who read may learn to prize more highly the inestimable gifts of sight and hearing.

MARY SWIFT LAMSON.

CONTENTS.

CHAPTER VII.

CHAPTER VIII.

CHAPTER IX.

CHAPTER X.

CHAPTER XI.

CHAPTER XII.

CHAPTER XIII.

CHAPTER XIV.

CHAPTER. XV.

CHAPTER XVI.

CHAPTER XVII.

LAURA BRIDGMAN.

CHAPTER I.

LAURA DEWEY BRIDGMAN was born Dec. 21, 1829, in Hanover, N. H. She was the child of Daniel and Harmony Bridgman. Her parents are described * as of —

"the average height, and though slenderly built, of sound health and good habits. The father's temperament inclined to the nervous, but he had a small brain ; while the mother had a very marked development of the nervous system, and an active brain, though not a large one.

"They were persons of good moral character, and had received about as much culture as is common in the rural districts of New Hampshire.

"The child inherited most of the physical peculiarities of the mother, with a dash of what, from want of a better name, is called the 'scrofulous temperament.' This temperament makes one very liable to certain diseases, but it gives great delicacy of fibre, and consequent sensibility. Laura had a physical organization like that of a delicate plant, — very liable to derange-

---

* Barnard's Am. Journal of Education, December, 1867 (article by Dr. S. G. Howe).

ment because very sensitive, also very difficult **as an** organization to bring to maturity, but promising great capacity and beauty."

During her infancy she was subject to severe convulsions, but at the age of eighteen months her health improved, and when two years old, she is described as being more active and intelligent than ordinary children. She had learned to speak a few words, and knew some of the letters of the alphabet. But her release from suffering was of short duration; for a month after, scarlet fever entered the family, which then consisted of three little girls. Her two older sisters died of the disease, and Laura's life long hung by a very slender thread. For seven weeks she was unable to swallow any solid food; both eyes and ears suppurated and discharged their contents, and sight and hearing were destroyed. Her eyes were very painful, and for five months she was kept in a darkened room.

The sense of smell was so nearly destroyed that it was useless, and she could scarcely distinguish between different articles of food by the taste : her only means of communication with the outer world was the touch. A year passed before she could walk without support, and two years before she was sufficiently strong to sit up all day.

At five years of age she had regained her strength, and her mind, which had been unim-

paired by all this bodily suffering, now hungered
for food. The long sickness had effaced the recollection of babyhood; the words once spoken
were long since forgotten; she had become dumb,
because she was deaf. She must begin life anew,
and her thirst for knowledge must be satisfied by
obtaining such information as one sense could
bring. Of everything she must feel, and all the
properties perceivable by that sense must be ascertained. As the mother moved about her various avocations, the child was always beside her,
the little hands felt every motion, and soon the
desire of imitation was developed. She was
taught to sew, to knit, and to braid. The only
way of communicating with her was by the simplest signs : extending the hand in a certain way
meant bread; raised to the lips as if tipping a
cup, drink; pushing — go; pulling — come; a pat
on the head expressed approval; on the back,
disapproval, etc. She was affectionate in disposition, but as she grew in strength and age, her
will developed, and restraint became more difficult. On her father devolved the unpleasant
task of compelling obedience. She had a friend
in an old man who loved her dearly, and of whom
she always in after life spoke with the greatest
affection. In his strong arms she delighted to be
carried, and with him, when able to walk, she
rambled through the fields and by the river-side,

taking pleasure in throwing stores into the water, though her eye could not watch them nor her ear hear their plashing.

Only one case similar to Laura's had ever been known in this country, and that was Julia Brace, who lost her senses of sight and hearing at four years of age, and who was living at this time at the Asylum for Deaf-Mutes, in Hartford, Conn. She had been taught to communicate to some extent, by signs only. Dr. S. G. Howe, director of the Institution for the Blind in Boston, had visited Julia, and had formed a theory for reaching a mind so enclosed. Hearing, soon after, of this little girl in New Hampshire, he went to see her, and persuaded the parents to place her under his charge.

She was brought to the Institution in Boston, Oct. 12, 1837, about two months before her eighth birthday.

Of the development of this theory and its application to her instruction, Dr. Howe has given brief accounts in his annual reports, but as the question most frequently asked is, " What was done first? " I have thought it desirable to obtain all possible information on that point.

For the interesting account which follows I am indebted to Mrs. L. H. Morton (Miss Drew), of Halifax, Mass., who assisted Dr. Howe in all these early lessons, and who continued to be

Laura's teacher for several years. She writes as follows : —

" Laura was a healthy little girl, with very fair complexion and light-brown hair ; and there was nothing in her appearance to distinguish her from the other little blind girls, except that she was more quiet and undemonstrative. This was, perhaps, because all were strangers to her. She first made the acquaintance of the matron, Mrs. Smith, to whom she seemed to be especially attracted, whose greetings would light up her face with smiles, while she returned her caresses with interest. She spent her time in knitting, and would take her work to Mrs. Smith if she dropped a stitch, and smile quietly as it was returned with a sign of approbation. At this time she uttered only a little pleasant noise ; but as she became better acquainted, this grew louder and very disagreeable.

" When I had been with her a few days, and she had become accustomed to being led about by me, I took her one morning to the nursery ; and having seated her by a table, Dr. Howe and myself commenced her first lesson. He had had printed, in the raised letters used by the blind, the names of many common objects, such as knife, fork, spoon, key, bed, chair, stove, door, etc., and had pasted some of the labels on the correspon ling articles. First we gave her the word, ' knife,' on the slip of paper, and moved her fingers over it, as the blind do in reading. Then we showed her the knife, and let her feel the label upon it, and made to her the sign which she was accustomed to use to signify likeness, viz , placing side by side the fore-

fingers of each hand. She readily perceived the simi-
larity of the two words.

" The same process was repeated with other articles.
This exercise lasted three quarters of an hour. She
received from it only the idea that some of the labels
were alike, and others unlike. The lesson was repeated
in the afternoon, and on the next day, and about the
third day she began to comprehend that the words on
the slips of paper represented the object on which they
were pasted. This was shown by her taking the word .
'chair' and placing it first upon one chair, and then upon
another, while a smile of intelligence lighted her hitherto
puzzled countenance, and her evident satisfaction
assured us that she had mastered her first lesson. In
succeeding lessons, the label having been given her, she
would search for the article, and having found it, place
it upon it. Then the operation was reversed, and having the article given, she found the proper label.

" Thus far she had studied the words as a whole, and
it was now desirable to have her form them herself from
their component letters. Mr. S. P. Ruggles. who had
charge of the printing department, was called upon to
construct a case of metal types. This contained four
sets of the alphabet, and afforded her much amusement
as well as profit. She seemed never to tire of setting
up the types to correspond with the printed words with
which she was already familiar. All the letters of one
alphabet were kept arranged in their proper order, while
she used the others. In less than three days she had
learned this order, as was found by taking all the types
from the case, and making a sign to her to rearrange
them, which she did without assistance.

" During the time of her earliest instruction, it was necessary to use many signs. These were laid aside, however, as soon as we had something better to supply their place. As a mark of approval, I stroked her hair or patted her upon the head ; of disapproval, knocked her elbow lightly.

" Whenever she overcame a difficulty, a peculiarly sweet expression lighted up her face, and we perceived that it grew daily more intelligent.

" It was nearly two months before any use was made of the manual alphabet. At this time Dr. Howe gave me a letter of introduction to Mr. George Loring, who was a deaf-mute, and a graduate from the Institution at Hartford. In one afternoon he taught me the alphabet, and the next day 1 began to teach it to Laura, showing her the position of the fingers to represent each of the types which she had been using.

" The method of teaching her new words afterwards was as follows : To let her examine an object, and then teach her its name by spelling it with my fingers. She placed her right hand over mine, so she could feel every change of position, and with the greatest anxiety, watched for each letter ; then she attempted to spell it herself ; and as she mastered the word, her anxiety changed to delight. Next she took her board, and arranged the types to spell the same word, and placed them near the object, to show that she understood it.

" She very soon perceived that spelling the words in this way was much more rapid, and attended with much less difficulty, than the old method with types, and immediately applied it practically. I shall never forget the first meal taken after she appreciated the use of the finger alphabet. Every article that she touched must have a name; and I was obliged to call some one to help me wait upon the other children, while she kept me busy in spelling the new words. Dr. Howe had been absent for some time, and on his return was much delighted with the progress she had made, and at once learned the manual alphabet himself.

" After she had learned a hundred or more common nouns, we began to teach her the use of verbs. The first were shut, open; shut door, open door, accompanying the spelling of the word by the act. In this way she learned those in constant use, and then we taught her adjectives, and the names of individuals. In a very short time she had learned the names of all our large family.

" After a year she began to learn to write. A pasteboard with grooved lines such as the blind use, was placed between the folds of the paper; a letter was pricked in stiff paper so that she might feel its shape, and then her right hand, holding the pencil, was guided to form it, the forefinger of the left hand following the point of the pencil, guiding the writing, and keeping the spaces between the letters. She did not learn to write well as quickly as many of the blind children.

" She was very social, and always wished to have some one sit beside her or walk with her, and she taught her little blind friends the finger alphabet.

" One day I was passing the door of the linen-room, and saw her standing upon a chair, examining the contents of an upper drawer. It contained pieces of ribbon and laces belonging to the matron. She took them out, felt of the smooth satin and the delicate lace, soliloquized with her fingers, and made a motion as if to appropriate them, then knocked her elbow (the sign of wrong), and after some hesitation replaced them. This was repeated several times, and then I went to her, and took her hand as if wishing to speak to her, when an expression of conscious guilt overspread her face. I made her understand by signs that she must not meddle with what did not belong to her. She said, ' Laura, wrong, no; Laura, right,' patting her own head, and showing me that she had not taken anything, but I knew that she had been under great temptation and had triumphed over it.

" I accompanied her on her first visit to her home in Hanover, in 1839. Her father met us in Lebanon, and as he took her hand she recognized him, and I taught her the word ' father.' She had seen her mother a year before, and had learned the word ' mother' at the time of her visit to the Institution. Before Laura could be persuaded to take off her cloak and bonnet after arriving at home, she took me over the whole house, showing me everything, and inquiring the names of things which she had not learned about in Boston. In an unfinished room were a loom and spinning-wheel. These she had seen (felt) her mother use, and was very anxious for their name. Then she led me to the bee-hive to know what that was.

" At this time she was very shy of gentlemen, and would hardly approach any one but Dr. Howe, and I thought she might repel her father and her old friend Mr. Tenny, but, on the contrary, she was much pleased to walk with him, as she had been in the habit of doing before she left home.

" She was anxious to have her mother talk with her, and began at once to teach her the alphabet.

" She seemed so happy to be at home that I feared she might object to return with me, but at the end of a fortnight she was quite willing to go, and left her mother very calmly."

CHAPTER II.

No regular journal of Laura's lessons was kept until June, 1840, but we find in the annual reports of Dr. Howe a summary of her progress from year to year, as well as a statement of her physical, mental, and moral condition.

At the close of the year 1838, when she had been sixteen months under instruction, he writes as follows : —*

"It has been ascertained beyond the possibility of doubt that she cannot see a ray of light, cannot hear the least sound, and never exercises her sense of smell, if she has any. Thus her mind dwells in darkness and stillness, as profound as that of a closed tomb at midnight. Of beautiful sights and sweet sounds and pleasant odors she has no conception ; nevertheless, she seems as happy and playful as a bird or a lamb ; and the employment of her intellectual faculties, or acquirement of a new idea, gives her a vivid pleasure, which is plainly marked in her expressive features. She never seems to repine, but has all the buoyancy and gaiety of childhood. She is fond of fun and frolic,

---

* Seventh Report of the Trustees of the New England Institution for the Blind.

and when playing with the rest of the children, her shrill laugh sounds loudest of the group.

When left alone, she seems very happy if she has her knitting or sewing, and will busy herself for hours : if she has no occupation, she evidently amuses herself by imaginary dialogues, or by recalling past impressions ; she counts with her fingers or spells out names of things which she has recently learned, in the manual alphabet of the deaf-mutes.   In this lonely self-communion she seems to reason, reflect, and argue ; if she spells a word wrong with the fingers of her right hand, she instantly strikes it with her left, as her teacher does, in sign of disapprobation ; if right, then she pats herself upon the head, and looks pleased.   She sometimes purposely spells a word wrong with the left hand, looks roguish for a moment and laughs, and then with the right hand strikes the left, as if to correct it.

" During the year she has attained great dexterity in the use of the manual alphabet of the deaf-mutes ; and she spells out the words and sentences which she knows. so fast and so deftly, that only those accustomed to this language can follow with the eye the rapid motion of her fingers.

" But wonderful as is the rapidity with which she writes her thoughts upon the air, still more so is the ease and accuracy with which she reads the words thus written by another, grasping their hand in hers, and following every movement of their fingers, as letter after letter conveys their meaning to her mind.   It is in this way that she converses with her blind playmates ; and nothing can more forcibly show the power of mind in forcing matter to its purpose, than a meeting between them. For if great talent and skill are necessary for two pantomimes to paint their thoughts and feelings by the movements of the body and the expression of the countenance, how much greater the difficulty when darkness shrouds them both, and the one can hear no sound !

" When Laura is walking through a passageway, with her hands spread before her, she knows instantly every one she meets, and passes them with a sign of recognition ; but if it be a girl of her own age, and especially if one of her favorites, there is instantly a bright smile of recognition and a twining of arms, a grasping of hands, and a swift telegraphing upon the tiny fingers, whose rapid evolutions convey the thoughts and feelings from the outposts of one mind to those of the other. There are questions and answers, exchanges of joy or sorrows, there are kissings and partings, just as between little children with all their senses.

" One such interview is a better refutation of the doctrine that mind is the result of sensation than folios of learned argument. If those philosophers who consider man as only the most perfect animal, and attribute his superiority to his senses, be correct, then a dog or a monkey should have mental power quadruple that of poor Laura Bridgman, who has but one sense.

" During this year, and six months after she had left home, her mother came to visit her, and the scene of their meeting was an interesting one.

" The mother stood some time, gazing with overflow-ing eyes upon her unfortunate child, who, all uncon-scious of her presence, was playing about the room.

Presently Laura ran against her, and at once began feeling of her hands, examining her dress, and trying to find out if she knew her; but not succeeding in this, she turned away as from a stranger, and the poor woman could not conceal the pang she felt at finding that her beloved child did not know her.

" She then gave Laura a string of beads which she used to wear at home, which were recognized by the child at once, who with much joy put them around her neck, and sought me eagerly, to say she understood the string was from her home.

" The mother now tried to caress her, but poor Laura repelled her, preferring to be with her acquaintances.

" Another article from home was now given her, and she began to look much interested; she examined the stranger much closer, and gave me to understand that she knew she came from Hanover. She even endured her caresses, but would leave her with indifference at the slightest signal. The distress of the mother was now painful to behold; for although she had feared that she should not be recognized, the painful reality of being treated with cold indifference by a darling child was too much for woman's nature to bear.

" After a while, on the mother's taking hold of her again, a vague idea seemed to flit across Laura's mind that this could not be a stranger; she therefore felt of her hands very eagerly, while her countenance assumed an expression of intense interest; she became very pale, and then suddenly red; hope seemed struggling with doubt and anxiety, and never were contending emotions more strongly painted upon the human face. At this moment of painful uncertainty, the mother

drew her close to her side, and kissed her fondly, when
at once the truth flashed upon the child, and all mis-
trust and anxiety disappeared from her face, as with an
expression of exceeding joy she eagerly nestled to the
bosom of her parent, and yielded herself to her fond
embraces.

"After this, the beads were all unheeded; the playthings which were offered to her were utterly disre-
garded; her playmates, for whom but a moment before
she gladly left the stranger, now vainly strove to pull
her from her mother; and though she yielded her
usual instantaneous obedience to my signal to follow
me, it was evidently with painful reluctance. She
clung close to me, as if bewildered and fearful; and
when, after a moment, I took her to her mother, she
sprang to her arms, and clung to her with eager joy.

"I had watched the whole scene with intense interest,
being desirous of learning from it all I could of the
workings of her mind; but I now left them to indulge,
unobserved, those delicious feelings which those who
have known a mother's love may conceive, but which
cannot be expressed.

"The subsequent parting between Laura and her
mother showed alike the affection, the intelligence, and
the resolution of the child, and was thus noticed at the
time: 'Laura accompanied her mother to the door,
clinging close to her all the way, until they arrived at
the threshold, where she paused, and felt around to
ascertain who was near her. Perceiving the matron,
of whom she is very fond, she grasped her with one
hand, holding on, convulsively, to her mother with the
other; and thus she stood for a moment, then she

dropped her mother's hand, put her handkerchief to her eyes, and turning round, clung, sobbing, to the matron, while her mother departed, with emotions as deep as those of her child."

At the end of the year 1839, after she had been twenty-eight months under instruction, the following report was made of her case : —*

" The intellectual improvement of this interesting being, and the progress she has made in expressing her ideas, are truly gratifying.

" Having mastered the manual alphabet of the deaf-mutes, and learned to spell readily the names of everything within her reach, she was then taught words expressive of positive qualities, as ' hardness,' ' softness'; and she learned to express quality by connecting the adjectives, ' hard ' or ' soft,' with the substantive ; though she generally followed what one would suppose to be the natural order in the succession of ideas, by placing the substantive first.

" It was found too difficult, however, then, to make her understand any general expression of quality, as ' hardness,' ' softness,' in the abstract. Indeed, this is a process of mind most difficult of performance to any, especially to deaf-mutes.

" Next she was taught those expressions of relation to place which she could understand. For instance, a ring was taken and placed *on* a box, then the words were spelt to her, and she repeated them from imitation. Then the ring was placed on a hat, and a sign

* Eighth Annual Report of the Trustees of Perkins Institution and Massachusetts Asylum for the Blind.

given her to spell. She spelt, ' ring on box'; but being checked, and the right words given, she immediately began to exercise her judgment, and, as usual, seemed intently thinking. Then the same was repeated with a bag, a desk, and a great many other things, until at last she learned that she must name the thing *on* which the article was.

" Then the same article was put *into* the box, and the words 'ring *in* box' given to her. This puzzled her for many minutes, and she made many mistakes; for instance, after she had learned to say correctly whether the ring was *on* or *in* a box, a drawer, a hat, a bucket, etc., if she were asked, where is house, or matron, she would say, *in* box. Cross-questioning, however, is seldom necessary to ascertain whether she really understands the force of the words she is learning, for when the true meaning dawns upon her mind, the light spreads to her countenance.

" In this case, the perception seemed instantaneous, and the natural sign by which she expressed it was peculiar and striking: she spelt *o-n*, then laid one hand *on* the other; then she spelt *i-n*, and enclosed one hand *within* the other.

" She easily acquired a knowledge and use of active verbs, especially those expressive of *tangible action*, as to walk, to run, to sew, to shake.

" At first, of course, no distinction could be made of mood and tense; she used the words in a general sense, and according to the order of her *sense of ideas*. Thus, in asking some one to give her bread, she would first use the word expressive of the leading idea, and say,

2

' Bread, give Laura.' If she wanted water, she would say, ' Water, drink, Laura.'

" Soon, however, she learned the use of the auxiliary verbs, of the difference of past, present, and future tense. For instance, here is an early sentence, ' Keller is sick ; when will Keller well ' ? The use of *be* she had not acquired.

" Having acquired the use of substantives, adjectives, verbs, prepositions, and conjunctions, it was thought time to make the experiment of trying to teach her to *write*, and to show her that she might communicate her ideas to persons not in contact with her.

" It was amusing to witness the mute amazement with which she submitted to the process, the docility with which she imitated every motion, and the per-severance with which she moved her pencil over and over again in the same track, until she could form the letter. But when, at last, the idea dawned upon her that by this mysterious process she could make other people understand what she thought, her joy was boundless.

" Never did a child apply more eagerly and joyfully to any task than she did to this ; and in a few months she could make every letter distinctly, and separate words from each other ; and she actually wrote, unaided, a legible letter to her mother, in which she expressed the idea of her being well, and of her expectation of her going home in a few weeks. It was, indeed, a very rude and imperfect letter, couched in the language which a prattling infant would use. Still it shadowed forth, and expressed to her mother, the ideas that were passing in her own mind.

laura will write
letter to mother
laura will ride wi
wit fa ther. laura
will make hurse
for mother laura
will sleep with
mother and father
mother will love
and kiss laura now
laura will carry
letter for mother
laura will go seewale
laura will go home.

" She is familiar with the processes of addition and subtraction in small numbers. Subtraction of one number from another puzzled her for a time; but by help of objects she accomplished it. She can count and conceive objects to about one hundred in number; to express an indefinitely great number, or more than she can count, she says, *hundred.* If she thought a friend was to be absent many years, she would say, *Will come hundred Sundays*, meaning weeks. She is pretty accurate in measuring time, and seems to have an intuitive tendency to do it. Unaided by the changes of night and day, by the light, or the sound of any timepiece, she nevertheless divides time pretty accurately.

" With the days of the week, and the week itself as a whole, she is perfectly familiar. For instance, if asked, What day will it be in fifteen days more? she readily names the day of the week. The day she divides by the commencement and end of school, by the recesses, and by the arrival of meal-times.

" Those persons who hold that the capacity of perceiving and measuring the lapse of time is an innate and distinct faculty of the mind, may deem it an important fact that Laura evidently can measure time so accurately as to distinguish between a half and whole note of music. Seated at the piano-forte, she will strike the notes in a measure like the following, quite correctly : —

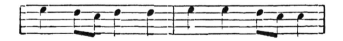

" Now it will be perceived that she must have clea] perception of lapse of time, in order to strike the two eighths at the right instant; for in the first measure they occur at the second beat, in the second measure at the third beat. She often asks questions which unfortunately cannot be satisfactorily answered to her, for it is painful to excite such a vivid curiosity as now exists in her mind, and then balk it. For instance, she once asked with much eagerness why one arrangement of letters was not as good as another to express the name of a thing; as why *t a c* should not express the idea of the animal, as well as *c a t.* This she expressed partly by signs and partly by words, but her meaning was perfectly clear; she was puzzled and wished an explanation.

" An extract from the diary kept by her instructor will give an idea of her manner of questioning : —

" *Dec. 3, 1839.* Spent one hour in giving Laura an idea of the meaning of the words 'left' and 'right.' She readily conceived that left hand, meant *her* left hand, but with difficulty generalized the term. At last, however, she caught the idea, and eagerly spelt the name of her arms, hands, fingers, feet, ears, etc., as they were touched, and named them, right or left, as might be : suddenly pausing, however, and looking puzzled, she put her finger on her *nose,* and asked if that were right or left ; thus she continually puzzles one ; but such is her eagerness to find out one's meaning, such a zealous co- operation is there on her part, that it is a delightful task to teach her.

" Uses to-day freely the prepositions *in* and *on ;* she says, ' teacher sit *in* sofa.' Do not dare to correct her ın such cases of anomalous usage of the preposition, but prefer to let her be in error than to shake her faith in a rule given : the corrections must be made by and by. The sofa having sides, she naturally says *in*.

" In her eagerness to advance her knowledge of words and to communicate her ideas she coins words, and is always guided by analogy. Sometimes her process of *word-making* is very interesting ; for instance, after some time spent in giving her an idea of the abstract meaning of *alone*, she seemed to obtain it, and understood that being *by one's self* was to be alone or *al-one*. She was told to go to her chamber, or school, or elsewhere, and return alone ; she did so, but soon after, wishing to go with one of the little girls, she strove to express her meaning thus : ' Laura go *al-two*.'

" The same eagerness is manifested in her attempts to define for the purpose of classification ; for instance, some one giving her the word ' bachelor' she came to her teacher for a definition ; she was taught that men who had wives were *husbands*, those who had none, *bachelors ;* when asked if she understood she said, ' man no have wife — bachelor ; Tenny — bachelor,' referring to an old friend of hers. Being told to define bachelor, she said, ' bachelor, no have wife, and smoke pipe.' Thus she considered the individual peculiarity of smoking, in one person, as a specific mark of the *species bachelor*.

" Then in order to test her knowledge of the word, it was said by her teacher, ' Tenny has got no wife, what is Tenny ?' She paused, and then said, ' Tenny is wrong.' The word ' widow ' being explained to her, a woman whose husband is dead, and being called upon to define, she said, ' Widow is woman, man dead and cold,' and eked out her meaning by sinking down, and dropping her hand, to signify *in the ground.*

" The last two words she added herself, they not having been in the definition ; but she instantly associates the idea of *coldness* and *burial* with death.

" She had touched a dead body before she came to the Institution.

" The following anecdote will give an idea of her fondness for teasing, or innocent fun or mischief. Her teacher, looking one day, unobserved, into the girls' play-room, saw three blind girls playing with the rocking horse. Laura was on the crupper, another in the saddle, and a third clinging on the neck, and they were all in high glee, swinging backward and forward as far as the rockers would roll. There was a peculiarly arch look in Laura's countenance, the natural language of sly fun. She seemed prepared to give a spring, and suddenly, when her end was lowest, and the others were perched high in the air, she sidled quickly off on to the floor, and down went the other end so swiftly as to throw the girls off the horse.

" This Laura evidently expected, for she stood a moment, convulsed with laughter, then ran eagerly forward with outstretched hands to find the girls, and almost screamed with joy. As soon, however, as she got hold of one of them, she perceived that she was hurt, and instantly her countenance changed, she seemed shocked and grieved, and after caressing and comforting her playmate, she found the other, and seemed to apologize by spelling the word ' wrong,' and caressing her.

" When she can puzzle her teacher, she is pleased, and often purposely spells a word wrong, with a playful look ; and if she catch her teacher in a mistake, she bursts into an ecstasy of laughter.

" With little girls of her own age, she is full of frolic and fun, and no one enjoys a game at *romps* more than Laura.

" She has the same fondness for dress, for ribbons, and for finery as other girls of her age, and as a proof that it arises from the same amiable desire of pleasing others, it may be remarked that whenever she has a new bonnet, or any article of dress, she is particularly desirous to go to meeting, or to go out with it. If people do not notice it, she directs their attention by placing their hands upon it.

" Generally she indicates her preference for such visitors as are the best dressed.

" It is interesting, in a physiological point of view, to know the effect of the deprivation of three senses on the remaining two.

" The sense of smell being destroyed, it seems a curious question whether the effect upon the organ of taste is general or particular, that is, whether the taste is blunted generally, and for all things alike, or whether one kind of sapidity is more affected than another. To ascertain this, some experiments have been tried, but as yet, not enough to enable one to state confidently the results in minute distinction. The general conclusions are these : —

" Acids seem to make vivid and distinct impressions upon the taste ; and she apparently distinguishes the different degrees of acidity better than of sweetness or bitterness. She can distinguish between wine, cider, and vinegar, better than substances like manna, liquorice, and sugar. Of bitters she seems to have less perception, or, indeed, hardly any; for on putting powdered rhubarb into her mouth, she called it *tea*, and on saying *no*, and telling her to taste *close*, she evidently did try to taste it, but still called it tea, and spit it out, but without any contortion or any indication of its being particularly disagreeable.

" Of course she has a repugnance to this kind of experiments, and it seems almost imposing upon her good-nature to push them very far.

" Those who are curious in the physiology of the taste know that the highest degree of *gusto*, or the acme of pleasure, is not obtained until just as the morsel has slipped over the glottis, and is on its way, beyond power of recall, down the œsophagus. This seems to be a wise precaution of nature to prevent the stomach being cheated of its due; for if the highest degree in pleasure of eating could be obtained without absolutely swallowing the morsel, the epicure could have an exhaustless source of pleasure, and need never degenerate into the *gourmand*.

" Some physiologists who have speculated upon this subject consider that this final climax of the pleasure of taste is produced by a fine aroma which, rising from the morsel and mounting up the fauces, pleasantly titillates the ramifications of the olfactory nerve. The fact that when we have a cold in the head, and the fauces are obstructed, the taste is blunted, seems to bear out this supposition; but from some observations on Laura,

one would be inclined to think that some other cause
must contribute to the effect.

"She appears to care less for the process of mastication than deglutition ; and probably it is only the necessity of mechanical trituration of foods which induces
her to go through with it, before hastening to the pleasant part of swallowing. Now, as the imperfection of
smell impairs the taste in the tongue and palate during
mastication, it should have the same effect in deglutition, supposing this theory to be correct ; but it seems
not to be so, else Laura would have little inducement
to swallow, save to fill a vacuity of stomach. Now it
seems doubtful whether the feeling of vacuity of stomach, strictly speaking, would show a child the road for
the food, or whether it would not be as likely to stuff
bread into its ear as into its mouth if it had no pleasurable sensation in tasting ; and further, if the pleasurable sensation did not increase, and tempt to deglutition,
it is doubtful whether hunger or vacuity of stomach
alone, would teach a child to swallow the chewed
morsel.

"On the whole, she seems to care less for eating
than most children of her age.

"With regard to the sense of touch it is very acute,
even for a blind person. It is shown remarkably in the
readiness with which she distinguishes persons. There
are forty inmates in the female wing, with all of whom
of course Laura is acquainted ; whenever she is walking
through the passage-ways, she perceives by the jar of
the floor or the agitation of the air that some one is
near her, and it is exceedingly difficult to pass her without being recognized. Her little arms are stretched

out, and the instant she grasps a hand, a sleeve, or even part of the dress, she knows the person and lets them pass on with some sign of recognition.

"The innate desire for knowledge, and the instinctive efforts which the human faculties make to exercise their functions, is shown most remarkably in Laura. Her tiny fingers are to her as eyes and ears and nose, and most deftly and incessantly does she keep them in motion. Like the feelers of some insects which are continually agitated, and which touch every grain of sand in the path, so Laura's arms and hands are continually in play ; and when she is walking with a person she not only recognizes everything she passes within touching distance ; but by continually touching her companion's hands she ascertains what he is doing. A person walking across a room while she had hold on his left arm, would find it hard to take a pencil out of his waistcoat pocket with his right hand, without her perceiving it.

" Her judgment of distances and of relations of place is very accurate ; she will rise from her seat, go straight towards a door, put out her hand just at the right time, and grasp the handle with precision.

"When she runs against a door which is shut, but which she expects to find open, she does not fret, but rubs her head and laughs, as though she perceived the ludicrous position of a person flat against a door trying to walk through it.

" The constant and tireless exercise of her feelers gives her a very accurate knowledge of everything about the house ; so that if a new article, a bundle, bandbox, or even a new book is laid anywhere in the apartments which she frequents, it would be but a short time before in her ceaseless rounds she would find it, and from something about it, she would generally discover to whom it belonged.

" She perceives the approach of persons by the undulations of the air striking her face, and she can distinguish the step of those who tread hard and jar the floor.

" At table, if told to be still, she sits and conducts herself with propriety; handles her cup, spoon, and fork like other children; so that a stranger looking at her would take her for a very pretty child with a green ribbon over her eyes.

" But when at liberty to do as she chooses, she is continually feeling of things, and ascertaining their size, shape, density, and use, asking their names and their purposes, going on with insatiable curiosity, step by step, towards knowledge.

" Thus doth her active mind, though all silent and darkling within, commune by means of her one sense with things external, and gratify its innate craving for knowledge by close and ceaseless attention.

" Qualities and appearances, unappreciable or unheeded by others, are to her of great significance and value; and by means of these her knowledge of external nature and physical relations will in time become extensive."

CHAPTER III.

In June, 1840, her teacher, Miss Drew, returned, after an absence of six months. From
her journal of the remainder of the year we quote
items of interest. Before commencing the summer term she accompanied Laura on a visit to
her parents. Her health was very delicate, and
she suffered much from pain in her side, which
she attributed entirely to the long journey. This
she expressed in the following words, which give
the reader a very good idea of her use of language
at this date: "When Laura did go to see mother,
ride did make Laura side ache ; horse was wrong, —
did not run softly." While at breakfast one day,
she asked, "Who did make egg?" Hen. "With
foot?" No. "Laura do love egg. Hen must
make more egg." June 20 she received her first
lesson in arithmetic on the metallic case used by
the blind. This is perforated with square holes,
and two square types are used to represent the
digits. The corner of one end is raised, and
represents 1, 3, 7, and 9, according to position in
the board or case. On the other end of the same

type is a diagonal line and a raised corner representing 2, 4, 6, 8. The second type has, on one
end. simply a diagonal line, representing 5 ; the
other end, which is flat, 0. She was delighted with
her lesson, as she always is with anything new ;
but it took several days to make her understand
the connection between the position of the type
in the aperture and its significance."

" *July 9.* She had learned to add a column of
figures amounting to thirty.

" For a month she was not well. and so excessively
nervous that her lessons were omitted.

" *Aug. 20.* A gentleman called to see Laura who
was going to Hartford. She had been told that there
was a person in the asylum there who was deaf, dumb,
and blind, and asked if she might send her a letter.
She wrote, ' Julia Brace cannot see and hear, — sorry,
— Laura is blind and deaf.'

" *Aug 22.* She was asked by her teacher to go to
the school-room to find a lead pencil, and told that she
did not· know on *which* desk it was. She returned
bringing the pencil, and said, ' Laura cannot find
which.' She had had several lessons upon the pronouns, I and you, and had used them properly, but
never had learned any others.

" *Aug. 24.* Gave her sentences introducing if, or,
which, and the past tense of the verbs come and go.

" *Aug. 26.* She was very impatient while writing
for company, and at last said, ' I do not want to write
for twenty ladies.'

" *Aug. 31.* Taught her the words Mr., Mrs., Miss.

She asked if she was Miss Laura. She uses the words
' me ' and ' my ' correctly to-day. If, by chance, she
converses with any one who uses proper names where
pronouns should be used, she looks very wise, and
knocks the person's elbow, and threatens to complain
of her to her teacher.

" *Sept. 2.* Her lesson was upon the formation of the
plural. She wishes to form them all by adding ' s,' but
quite dislikes the idea that some nouns ending in ' ey '
must have an ' s ' while others change to ' ies.'

" *Sept. 7.* Laura came to me saying, ' Dog did come
in school-room. Susan did strike dog, — dog was
wrong to come in school-room,' and then she laughed
aloud at the idea of a dog coming to school. That I
might see what reply she would make, I told her she
must teach the dog. She asked, ' Can dog learn? Can
dog talk with fingers?' and added, laughing heartily,
' Dog has no fingers.'

" *Sept. 8.* Dr. R. visited the school to-day and was
much interested in Laura, but it was impossible to make
her converse about anything. She wrote badly, and
seemed anxious to go away to play. In the afternoon,
I told her I was sorry she was not good when Dr. R.
was here; she very adroitly changed the subject, asking, ' Has Dr. R. got little cow in home?'

" *Sept. 11.* A visitor at the school said he had a
deaf and dumb boy at home. I repeated it to Laura
thus, ' Man has little boy *who* cannot see and hear.'
She wrote as a specimen of her writing, ' I am sorry
who cannot see and hear. I am blind and deaf.' She
probably thought that ' who ' was the name of the boy.

" *Nov. 5.* Find it difficult to make her comprehend

the use of it, they, them. Speaking of a lady who has died, and whom she saw in Hanover two years ago, she said, ' Will Mrs. M. come back when sun is warm? where is Mrs. M.? are you sorry not to see Mrs. M.?'

" *Nov. 6.* She asked, ' Where are flies gone?' I told her the cold made the flies die. ' Will flies come when warm?' Yes ' I am sorry lady will not come when warm.'

" *Nov. 11.* In Laura's lesson in arithmetic I told her she was ' adding.' She thought a moment, and said, ' I added yesterday and counted.' I said, ' I will tell doctor you can add very good.' 'When will you tell him?' ' After dinner, if I see him.' She immediately said, ' If he will not go to Boston,' showing that she applies *if* correctly at last. In one of her sums the answer consisted of four figures, and she did not know the name of thousands. I explained that one thousand was the same as ten hundred, and she read the number 1875, ' ten hundred, and eight hundred, and seventy-five.'

" *Nov. 18.* Laura has lately reported many misdeeds of her playmates. To-day she came to say, ' Olive pinched very hard. You must knock Olive very much hard, she pinched and was wrong.'

" *Nov. 29.* Our little blind pupil, Adeline, breathed her last this afternoon. Her death, although every hour expected, came like a chill upon all our hearts, for she was beloved by us all. The little girls of her own age were much affected Laura was puzzled; she could not understand the mystery of death, but she seemed grieved, and asked, ' Will Adeline's mother cry and be very sorry? Is she cold and stiff? What is die?'

" *Dec. 2.* Laura was much grieved that she could not go to Cambridge ' to see Adeline,' and asked many questions, which it was impossible to answer. ' Where is Adeline? can she breathe? when will she be well?'

" *Dec. 12.* Laura has been confined to her bed for several days, but was able to sit up to-day. She highly enjoys being comfortably sick, and it delights her to sit in a rocking-chair with a shawl wrapped around her, and then to be served with such delicacies as she thinks proper for an invalid, as roasted apple, cracker toast, etc.

" *Dec. 30.* She was in the dining-room closet, where there were some apples, and told the little girl who was with her she wanted an apple. Elizabeth gave her one, but she refused it, and said, ' No, Elizabeth must ask Mrs. Smith if she can give me apple.' 1 have observed frequently that she will not take anything that she knows does not belong to her. At one time a piece of candy lay upon my table; she touched it accidentally, took it up, and made a sign that she would eat it, then laid it down again, and knocked her elbow as if she had done wrong to take it up, and shook her head to signify it was not hers."

In the Ninth Annual Report to the Trustees at the close of the year 1840, Dr. Howe writes : —

" I shall now notice such of the phenomena that I have remarked in her case during the last year, as seem most striking and important.

" Her health has been very good. She has not grown much in height, but her frame has filled out.

" A perceptible change has taken place in the size

and shape of her head ; and although unfortunately the measurement taken two years ago has been mislaid, every one who has been well acquainted with her notices a marked increase in the size of the forehead. She is now just eleven years old ; her height is four feet four inches and seven tenths. Her head measures twenty inches and eight tenths in circumference, in a line drawn around it, and passing over the prominences of the parietal and those of the frontal bones ; above this line the head rises one inch and one tenth, and is broad and full. The measurement is four inches from one orifice of the ear to the other ; and from the occipital spine to the root of the nose, it is seven inches.

" Nothing has occurred to indicate the slightest perception of light or sound, or any hope of it ; and although some of those who are much with her suppose that her smell is more acute than it was, even this seems very doubtful.

" It is true that she sometimes applies things to her nose, but often it is merely in imitation of the blind children about her ; and it is unaccompanied by that peculiar lighting up of the countenance which is observable whenever she discovers any new quality in an object.

" It was stated in the first report that she could perceive very pungent odors, such as that of cologne ; but it seemed to be as much by the irritation it produced upon the mucous membrane of the nares as by any impression upon the olfactory nerve.

" It is clear that the sensation cannot be pleasurable, nor even a source of information to her respecting physical qualities ; for such is her eagerness to gain
3

this information, that could smell serve her, she would exercise it incessantly.

" Those who have seen Julia Brace, or any other deaf-blind person, would hardly fail to observe how quickly they apply everything which they feel to the nose, and how, by this incessant exercise, the smell becomes almost incredibly acute. Now with Laura this is not the case; she seldom puts a new thing to her nose, and when she does, it is mechanically, as it were, and without any interest.

" Her sense of touch has evidently improved in acuteness; for she now distinguishes more accurately the different undulations of the air, or the vibrations of the floor, than she did last year. She perceives very readily when a door is opened or shut, though she may be sitting at the opposite side of the room. She perceives also the tread of persons upon the floor.

" Her mental perceptions, resulting from sensation, are much more rapid than they were, for she now perceives, by the slightest touch, qualities and conditions of things, similar to those she had formerly to feel long and carefully for. So with persons; she recognizes her acquaintances in an instant, by touching their hands or their dress; and there are probably fifty individuals who, if they should stand in a row, and hold out each a hand to her, would be recognized by that alone

" The memory of these sensations is very vivid, and she will readily recognize a person whom she has thus once touched. Many cases of this kind have been noticed; such as a person shaking hands with her, and making a peculiar pressure with one finger, and repeating this on his second visit after a lapse of many months, being instantly known by her. She has been known to recognize persons whom she had thus simply shaken hands with but once, after a lapse of six months.

" This is not more wonderful, indeed, than that one should be able to recall impressions made upon the mind through the organ of sight, as when we recogniz? a person of whom we had but one glimpse a year be fore ; but it shows the exhaustless capacity of those organs of sense which the Creator has bestowed, as it were in reserve against accidents, and which we usually allow to live unused and unvalued.

" The progress which she has made in intellectual acquirements can be fully appreciated by those only who have seen her frequently. The improvement, however, is made evident by her greater command of language, and by the conception which she now has of the force of parts of speech which last year she did not use in her simple sentences ; for instance, of pronouns, which she has begun to use within six months. This will be seen by an extract from the diary of one of her teachers written last month, Dec. 18 : ' To-day Laura asked me, " What is voice ? " I told her as well as I could that it was the noise people make when they talk with their mouths. She then said, " I do not voice." I said, " Can you talk with your mouth ? " *Answer :* " No." " Why ? " " Because I am very deaf and dumb." " Can you see ? " " No, because I am blind, I did not talk with fingers when I came with my mother, doctor did teach me on fork." " What was on fork ? " I told her paper was fixed on forks. She

then said, " I did learn to read much with types, doctor did teach me in nursery.   Drusilla was very sick all
over." '

" The words here given (and indeed in all cases) are
precisely as she used them ; for great care is taken to
note them at the time of utterance.   It will be observed
that she uses the pronoun, personal and possessive ;
and so ready is she to conceive the propriety of it, and
the impropriety of her former method, that upon my
recently saying, ' Doctor will teach Laura,' she eagerly
shook my arm to correct me, and told me to say, ' *I*
will teach *you*.'   She is delighted when she can catch
any one in an error like this ; and she shows her sense
of the ludicrous by laughter, and gratifies her innocent
self-esteem by displaying her knowledge

" She easily learned the difference between the singular and plural form, but was inclined for some time
to apply the rule of adding *s*, universally.   For instance, at her first lesson she had the words, *arm, arms,
hand, hands*, etc. ; then being asked to form the plural
of box, she said boxs, and for a long time she would
form the plural by the general rule, as lady, ladys, etc.

" One of the girls had the mumps ; Laura learned
the name of the disease ; and soon after she had it herself, but she had the swelling only on one side ; and
some one saying, ' You have got the mumps,' she replied
quickly, ' No, I have mump.'

" With pronouns she had very little difficulty.   It
was thought best at first to talk with her as one does
with an infant ; and she learned to reply in the same
way.   ' Laura want water, give Laura water ' ; but she
readily learned to substitute the pronoun, and now says,

' Give me water. I want water,' etc. Indeed, she will
not allow persons to address her in the third person,
but instantly corrects them, being proud to show her
knowledge.

" She learned the difference between present and
past tense the last year, but made use of the auxilia-
ries; during this year she has learned the method of
inflecting the verb. In this process too her perfect
simplicity rebukes the clumsy irregularities of our language. She learned, jump, jumped, walk, walked, etc.,
until she had an idea of the mode of forming the imperfect tense, but when she came to the word *see*, she
insisted that it should be *seed* in the imperfect, and
after this, upon going down to dinner, she asked if it
was *eat, eated*, but being told it was *ate*, she seemed to
try to express the idea that this transposition of letters
was not only wrong but ludicrous, for she laughed
heartily.

" The eagerness with which she followed up these
exercises was very delightful; and the pupil, teasing
the teacher for more words, is in pleasing contrast with
the old method, where all the work was on one side,
and where the coaxing and scolding and birchen appli-
ances to boot, often failed to force an idea into the
mind in the proper shape. But Laura is always ready
for a lesson, and generally has prepared, beforehand,
a number of questions to put to her teacher; for
instance, when she was learning past tenses, she came
one morning with fourteen verbs, of which she knew
the present form, to ask for the imperfect.

" The most recent exercises have been upon those
words which would require attention to one's own

mental operations, such as remember, forget, expect, hope, etc.

"Greater difficulties have been experienced in these than in her former lessons; but they have been so far surmounted that she uses many words of this kind with a correct perception of their meaning.

"The day after her first lesson on the words, 'I remember' and 'I forget,' this memorandum was made of her second lesson on the same words. *Question:* ' What do you remember you did do last Sunday?' *Answer:* ' I remember not to go to meeting' (meaning that she did not go to meeting). *Question:* ' What do you remember you did on Monday?' *Answer:* ' To walk in streets, on snow' (this was correct). *Question:* ' What do you remember you did in vacation?' *Answer:* ' What is vacation?' This was a new word to her. She had been accustomed to say, ' When is no school,' or, ' When girls go home.' The word being explained, she said, ' 1 remember to go to Halifax' (meaning that she did go to Halifax, which was true). ' What do you remember you did in vacation before?' *Answer:* ' To play with Olive, Maria, and Lydia' (these were the girls who had been her companions).

"Wishing to make her use the word 'forget,' I pushed the questions back to periods which she could not recall. I said, ' What did you do when you were a little baby?' She replied, laughing, ' I did cry,' and made the sign of tears running down her cheeks.

"' What did you *say?*' No answer. ' Did you talk with fingers?' ' No' (very decidedly). ' Did you talk with mouth?' A pause. ' What did you say with mouth?'

' I forget.' I then quickly let her know that this was the proper word, and of the same force as ' I do not remember.' Thinking this to be a good opportunity of testing her recollection of her infancy, many questions were put to her; but all that could be learned satisfactorily was that she could recollect lying on her back, and in her mother's arms, and having medicines poured down her throat, or, in her own words, ' I remember mother to give me medicines' (making the signs of lying down and of pouring liquids down the throat).

" It was not until after she had learned a few words of this kind that it was possible to carry her mind backwards to her infancy; and to the best of my judgment, she has no recollection of any earlier period than the long and painful illness in which she lost her senses. She seems to have no recollection of any words of prattle which she might have learned in the short respite which she enjoyed from bodily suffering.

" Thus far, her progress in the acquisition of language has been such as one would infer, *a priori*, from philosophical considerations; and the successive steps have been nearly such as Monboddo supposed were taken by savages in the formation of their language.

" But it shows clearly how valuable language is, not only for the *exp·ession* of thought, but for aiding mental development and exercising the higher intellectual faculties.

" When Laura first began to use words, she evidently had no idea of any other use than to express the individual existence of things, as book, spoon, etc. The sense of touch had, of course, given her an idea of their existence, and of their individual characteristics;

but one would suppose that specific differences would
have been suggested to her also ; that is, that in feeling
of many books, spoons, etc., she would have reflected
that some were large, some small, some heavy, some
light, and been ready to use words expressive of the
specific and generic character. But it would seem not
to have been so, and her first use of the words great,
small, heavy, etc., was to express merely individual
peculiarities : *great book* was to her the double name
of a particular book ; *heavy stone* was one particular
stone ; she did not consider those terms as expressive
of *sub tantive* specific differences, or any differences of
quality ; the words *great* and *heavy* were not considered
abstractly, as the name of a general quality, but they
were blended in her mind with the name of the objects
in which they existed. At least such seemed to me to
be the case, and it was not until some time after, that
the habit of abstraction enabled her to apply words of
generic signification in their proper way.

" This view is confirmed by the fact that when she
learned that persons had both individual and family
names, she supposed that the same rule must apply to
inanimate things, and asked earnestly what was the
other name for chair, table, etc.

" Several of the instances which have been quoted
will show her disposition to form her words by rule, and
to admit of no exceptions ; having learned to form the
plurals by adding *s*, the imperfect by adding *ed*, etc.,
she would apply this to every new noun or verb, consequently the difficulty hitherto has been greater, and her
progress slower, than it will be, for she has mastered
the most common words, and these seem to be the ones

that have been the most broken up by the rough colloquial usage of unlettered people.

The notice of her intellectual progress has thus far
related to the acquisition of language, and this, to her,
was the principal occupation ; other children learn language by mere imitation and without effort ; she has to
ask by a slow method the name of every new thing ;
other children use words which they do not understand,
but she wishes to know the force of every expression.
Her knowledge of language, however, is no criterion of
her knowledge of things, nor has she been taught mere
words.   She is like a child placed in a foreign country,
where one or two persons only know her language, and
she is constantly asking of them the names of the
objects around her.

The moral qualities of her nature have also developed
themselves more clearly.   She is remarkably correct in
her deportment, and few children of her age evince so
much sense of propriety in regard to appearance.
Never, by any possibility, is she seen out of her room
with her dress disordered ; and if, by chance, any spot
of dirt is pointed out to her on her person, or any little
rent in her dress, she discovers a sense of shame, and
hastens to remove it.

" She is never discovered in an attitude or an action
at which the most fastidious would revolt, but is remarkable for neatness, order, and propriety.

" There is one fact which is hard to explain in any
way : it is the difference of her deportment to persons of
different sex.   This was observable when she was only
seven years old.   She is very affectionate, and when
with her friends of her own sex she is constantly cling-

ing to them, and often kissing and caressing them ; and
when she meets with strange ladies, she very soon becomes familiar, examines very freely their dress, and
readily allows them to caress her.   But with those of
the other sex it is entirely different, and she repels every
approach to familiarity.   She is attached, indeed, to
some, and is fond of being with them ; but she will not
sit upon their knees, for instance, or allow them to take
her around the waist, or submit to those innocent famil-
iarities which it is common to take with children of her
age.

" She seems to have, also, a remarkable degree of
conscientiousness for one of her age ; she respects the
rights of others, and will insist upon her own.

" She is fond of acquiring property, and seems to
have an idea of ownership of things which she has long
since laid aside, and no longer uses.   She has never
been known to take anything belonging to another : and
never but in one or two instances to tell a falsehood,
and then only under strong temptation.   Great care,
indeed, has been taken not to terrify her by punishment, or to make it so severe as to tempt her to avoid
it by duplicity, as children so often do.

" When she has done wrong, her teacher lets her
know that she is grieved, and the tender nature of the
child is shown by the ready tears of contrition and
the earnest assurances of amendment with which she
strives to comfort those whom she has pained.

" When she has done anything wrong, and grieved her
teacher, she does not strive to conceal it from her little
companions, but communicates it to them, tells them
' it is wrong,' and says, ' —— cannot love wrong girl.'

" When she has anything nice given to her, she is particularly desirous that those who happen to be ill, or afflicted in any way, should share with her, although they may not be those whom she particularly loves in other circumstances ; nay, even if it be one whom she dislikes. She loves to be employed in attending the sick, and is most assiduous in her simple attentions and tender and endearing in her demeanor.

" It has been remarked in former reports that she can distinguish different degrees of intellect in others, and that she soon regarded, almost with contempt, a new-comer, when, after a few days, she discovered her weakness of mind. This unamiable part of her character has been more strongly developed during the past year.

" She chooses for her friends and companions those children who are intelligent, and can talk best with her ; and she evidently dislikes to be with those who are deficient in intellect, unless, indeed, she can make them serve her purposes, which she is evidently inclined to do. She takes advantage of them, and makes them wait upon her, in a manner that she knows she could not exact of others, and in various ways she shows her Saxon blood.

" She is fond of having other children noticed and caressed by the teachers, and those whom she respects ; but this must not be carried too far, or she becomes jealous. She wants to have her share, which, if not the lion's, is the greater part ; and if she does not get it, she says, ' My mother will love me.'

" Her tendency to imitation is so strong that it leads her to actions which must be entirely incomprehensible to her, and which can give her no other pleasure than the gratification of an internal faculty. She has been known to sit for a half an hour, holding a book before her sightless eyes, and moving her lips, as she has observed ' seeing people ' do when reading.

" She one day pretended that her doll was sick, and went through all the motions of tending it and giving it medicine; she then carefully put it to bed, and placed a bottle of hot water to its feet, laughing all the time most heartily. When I came home she insisted upon my going to see it, and feel its pulse; and when I told her to put a blister to its back, she seemed to enjoy it amazingly, and almost screamed with delight.

" Her social feelings and her affections are very strong; and when she is sitting at work, or at her studies, by the side of one of her little friends, she will break off from her task, every few moments, to hug and kiss her with an earnestness and warmth that is touching to behold.

" When left alone, she occupies and apparently amuses herself, and seems quite contented; and so strong seems to be the natural tendency of thought to put on the garb of language that she often soliloquizes in the *finger language*, slow and tedious as it is. But it is only when alone that she is quiet; for if she becomes sensible of the presence of any one near her, she is restless until she can sit close beside them, hold their hand, and converse with them by signs.

" She does not cry from vexation and disappointment, like other children, but only from grief. If she receives a blow by accident, or hurts herself, she laughs and jumps about, as if trying to drown the pain by muscular action. If the pain is severe, she does not go to her teachers or companions for sympathy, but on the contrary, tries to get away by herself, and then seems to give vent to a feeling of spite by throwing herself about violently, and roughly handling whatever she gets hold of.

" Twice only have tears been drawn from her by the severity of pain ; and then she ran away, as if ashamed of crying for an accidental injury. But the fountain of her tears is by no means dried up, as is seen when her companions are in pain or her teacher is grieved.

" In her intellectual character, it is pleasing to observe an insatiable thirst for knowledge and a quick perception of the relation of things.

" In her moral character it is beautiful to behold her continual gladness, her keen enjoyment of existence, her expansive love, her unhesitating confidence, her sympathy with suffering, her conscientiousness, truthfulness, and hopefulness."

We return to the journal of Miss Drew.

" *Jan. 13, 1841.* While Laura was playing with Lydia and Sophia, I told her to go to her room and brush her hair ' very quick,' and come to me. She refused at first. I insisted, and she went up stairs in a pet. In a little while she came into the school-room with Sarah, and looked very anxious. Sarah said she had told the little girls in the parlor that she could not go to school because Miss Drew was gone to Boston, and she came down with her to inquire if I were gone. When Laura took my hand she looked very pale, then red. I asked her what she did. She said, ' I did tell Louisa you were gone to Boston.' ' Why did you tell

her so?' 'Because I was very wrong and did say lie.'
She then attempted to justify herself, and asked, 'Why
did you tell me to go from Sophia?' I told her I
wished her to braid her hair. 'I did not want to go.'
Here the Doctor came in and she colored immediately.
He asked her what she had done. She said, 'I did
tell lie.' After he had left her I talked with her some
time and she seemed much grieved, and said, 'I am
sorry. I will be good and will not tell lie any more.'

"*Jan. 25.* Laura struck one of the little girls
against whom she has always an aversion, and after
repentance and forgiveness, she said, 'I will go home
and come no more.' I asked why. 'Because I cannot
be good in Boston.' I said, 'Your mother will be sorry
if you are naughty.' 'My mother will love me.' 'Yes,
but she will be sorry.' I asked her if she was sorry she
came to Boston. 'No, because I can (could) not talk
with fingers when I came with my father and mother.'
'If you go home and come no more, you can talk with
no one with fingers.' 'My mother will talk *little slow.*'

"P. M. I endeavored to overcome Laura's prejudices
against Olive, and tried to make her understand that
Olive was as good as she was. I said to her, 'You must
love Olive, and walk with her, and teach her to talk
with fingers.' She burst into a loud laugh, and said,
'Olive cannot learn to talk with fingers; her fingers
are very stiff. She cannot make good letters.' And
then she made a letter with her own fingers in a very
awkward manner to show me what might be expected
from her.

"*Feb. 6.* The crowd has become so great at the
monthly exhibitions, and presses so closely about

Laura, that we are obliged to surround her desk by settees, thus making a little enclosure and protecting her. Our first trial of the arrangement was to-day, and Laura was quite displeased with it. She asked, ' Are ladies afraid of me?' thinking that it was made for the people rather than for her **own good.**"

CHAPTER IV.

On Feb. 16, 1841, a deaf, dumb, and blind girl named Lucy Reed was brought to the Institution from Derby, Vt. She was at once an object of great interest to Laura, who was very anxious that she should be taught to talk with her. She was fourteen years of age, had never been controlled, and for a long time violently resisted all efforts to approach her, but she seemed to understand that Laura was like herself, and was attracted to her. Under date of April 14, Miss Drew records her first success after two months of daily effort.

" I tried to teach Lucy to spell the word 'fig' with her fingers, and succeeded in doing so after much trouble ; she would not do it, however, a second time, although she seemed very desirous of having the fig."

A week later she relates the following incident.

" I took a fork and gave her the letters, f-o-r-k. She was very indifferent, and manifested unwillingness to do what I wished her to, but she made the letters once. Presently Laura came in with some figs. I told her she must give Lucy one. She said, ' Lucy must spell fig before I give it to her.' She went to her and showed her the fig, and then spelled it very slowly on her own hand, then made signs to her make the letters herself. This Lucy would not do at first, but Laura persevered, and by signs made her understand that she might have the fig if she would spell it, and made the letters again on her own hand. and again made signs to her to make them herself. At last Lucy found that Laura was in earnest, and she spelled the word f-i-g. Laura then patted her on head and cheek, and seemed to be perfectly delighted that she had accomplished so much."

After this we often taught Lucy at the same time with Laura, when giving the latter a lesson which did not require undivided attention. This was a trial of her patience, and it was necessary to remind her how much she ought to pity Lucy, in order to reconcile her to the arrangement. It was merely the development of the same feeling we so often perceive in the family, when the little child finds itself supplanted by the new-born baby. Lucy remained with us only a few months, and the occasional references in the notes which follow will show Laura's interest in her.

At this point in Laura's history, June, 1841, my own notes commence. I had entered the Institution a year previous, as special teacher for Joseph Smith, a young blind man who was preparing for Harvard College.

Laura always made the acquaintance of every member of the family, and soon discovered me,

4

and taught me to use the manual alphabet. In August, Dr. Howe requested me to devote an hour daily to conversation with her. My remembrance of those early lessons is very limited, and no notes of them have been preserved. The difficulties encountered in teaching her comparison are, however, indelibly impressed upon my mind. At the close of the third week's work on this subject alone, I felt that I had exhausted all my own resources, and went to Dr. Howe for assistance. He dismissed me with the suggestion that I persevere, and in a day or two after, we triumphed. Perhaps this may be accounted for, in part, by my inexperience, as I was only eighteen, and just out of school, but the subsequent study of the development of other children convinces me that most of them meet the same difficulties, and that they are only overcome by much practice.

After a child has acquired a good use of language, the question, "Which do you like better, an apple or an orange?" will be answered by naming the object which happens to be mentioned last; reverse the order of the question, and the answer will be reversed.

When in the kitchen one day, Laura put her hand upon a turkey and asked what it was. She was told it was a dead bird. Some time afterward she asked of what the meat she was eating was made, and was told it was cow. This was a new revelation to her, and she refused to eat any meat for a number of weeks. We regretted it and said all we could to persuade her, for she was not strong, and it was thought a very necessary article of diet for her. Whether she perceived she was not as well in consequence we do not know, but she at length returned to it of her own accord, and we thought it unwise to make further conversation about it.

My journal entries from this time to May, 1845, were made daily, and begin as follows : —

June 8, 1841. Laura is not quite satisfied with her arithmetic lesson because I was teaching Lucy Reed at the same time. She finds much difficulty in doing her examples in subtraction ; but was made happy at last, because she detected me in a mistake.

June 9. Allowed her to converse instead of the arithmetic lesson, which always pleases her. Asked her questions that would lead to answers introducing the past tenses of verbs, and found them very correct. Several times she recalled a wrong word, correcting it herself before I alluded to it. When talking about bathing, she said, "Did you walk very weak in water? Water is very strong. Who made water?"

Referred her to Dr. Howe for a reply. In explanation of this, and in justice to myself, it is necessary for me to state that when Dr. Howe requested me to teach Laura, he expressed the wish that I should not converse with her on anything which should lead to religious subjects, but that I would refer her to him for answers to all questions tending in that direction, as he reserved to himself that part of her education.

In Appendix A to the Ninth Annual Report to the Trustees, which was written six months previous to this date, Dr. Howe gives his views on the subject of her religious teaching : —

" No religious feeling, properly so called, has developed itself; nor is it yet time, perhaps, to look for it ; but she has shown a disposition to respect those who have power and knowledge, and to love those who have goodness ; and when her perceptive faculties shall have taken cognizance of the operations of nature, and she shall be accustomed to trace effects to their causes, then may her veneration be turned to Him who is almighty, her respect to him who is omniscient, and her love to him who is all goodness and love !

" Until then, I shall not deem it wise, by premature effort, to incur the risk of giving her ideas of God which would be alike unworthy of his character and fatal to her peace.

" I should fear that she might personify Him in a way too common with children, who clothe him with unworthy, and sometimes grotesque, attributes, which their subsequently developed reason condemns, but strives in vain to correct.

" I am almost invariably questioned by intelligent visitors of the Institution about my opinion of her moral nature, and by what theory I can account for such and such phenomena ; and as many pious people have questioned me respecting her religious nature, I will here state my views.

" There seem to have been in this child no innate ideas or innate moral principles; that is, in the sense in which Locke, Condillac, and others consider those terms. But there are innate intellectual *dispositions;* and moreover, innate moral *dispositions*, not derived, as many metaphysicians suppose, from the exercise of intellectual faculties, but as independent in their existence as the intellectual dispositions themselves.

" I shall be easily understood when I speak of innate *dispositions*, in contradistinction to innate ideas, by those who are at all conversant with metaphysics; but as this case excites peculiar interest, even among children, I may be excused for explaining.

" We have no innate ideas of color, of distance, etc. ; were we blind, we never could conceive the idea of color, nor understand how light and shade could give knowledge of distance; but we might have the innate disposition, or internal adaptation, which enables us to perceive color, and to judge of distance; and were the organ of sight suddenly to be restored to healthy action, we should gradually understand the natural language, so to call it, of light; and soon be able to judge of distance, by reason of *our innate disposition or capacity.*

" So much for an intellectual perception. As an example of a moral perception, it may be supposed, for instance, that we have no innate idea of God, but that we have an innate disposition, or adaptation, not only to recognize, but to adore him; and when the idea of a God is presented, we embrace it, because we have that internal adaptation which enables us to do so.

" If the idea of a God were innate, it would be uni versal and identical, and not the consequential effect of the exercise of causality; it would be impossible to present him under different aspects. He would not be regarded as Jupiter, Jehovah, Brahma; we could not make different people clothe him with different attributes, any more than we could make them consider two and two to make three, or five, or anything but four.

" But on the other hand, if we had no *innate disposition* to receive the idea of a God, then could we never have conceived one, any more than we can conceive of time without a beginning; then would the most incontrovertible evidence to man of God's existence have been wanting, viz., the internal evidence of his own nature.

" Now, it does appear to me very evident, from the phenomena manifested in Laura's case, that she has innate moral dispositions and tendencies, which, though developed subsequently (in the order of time) to her intellectual faculties, are not dependent upon them, nor are they manifested with a force proportionate to that of her intellect.

" According to Locke's theory, the moral qualites and faculties of this child should be limited in proportion to the limitation of her senses, for he derives moral principles from intellectual dispositions, which alone he considers to be innate. He thinks moral principles must be *proved*, and can only be so by an exercised intellect.

" Now, the *sensations* of Laura are very limited; acute as is her touch, and constant as is her exercise of it, how vastly does she fall behind others of her age in the amount of sensations which she experiences, how limited is the range of her thought, how infantile is she in the exercise of her intellect! But her moral qualities, her moral sense, are remarkably acute; few children are so affectionate, or so scrupulously conscientious, few are so sensible of their own rights or regardful of the rights of others.

" Can any one suppose, then, that without innate moral dispositions, such effects could have been produced solely by moral lessons? for even if they could have been given to her, would they not have been seed sown upon barren ground? Her moral sense and her conscientiousness seem not at all dependent upon any intellectual perception; they are not perceived, indeed, or understood, — they are *felt*, and she may feel them even more strongly than most adults.

" These observations will furnish an answer to another question, which is frequently put concerning Laura: can she be taught the existence of God, her dependence upon, and her obligations to him?

" The answer may be inferred from what has gone before, — that, if there exists in her mind (and who can doubt that it does?) the innate capacity for the perception of this great truth, it can probably be developed, and become an object of intellectual perception and firm belief.

" I trust, too, that she can be made to conceive of future existence, and to lean upon the hope of it, as an anchor to her soul in those hours when sickness and approaching death shall arouse to fearful activity the instinctive love of life which is possessed by her in common with all.

"But to effect this, to furnish her with a guide through life and a support in death, much is to be done, and much is to be avoided.

" None but those who have seen her engaged in the task, and have witnessed the difficulty of teaching her the meaning of such words as *remember, hope, forget, expect*, will conceive the difficulties in her way; but they, too, have seen her unconquerable resolution, and her unquenchable thirst for knowledge; and they will not condemn as visionary such pleasing anticipations."

We continue the extracts from the journal : —

June 15. Laura succeeded in doing several examples in subtraction very well. For the last one under this rule gave her one with fifteen figures in the minuend. She said, " Sum is very long, like Halifax."

She thought her journey to that place took a long time, hence the comparison. Some time ago she read in " The Child's Book ' (printed in raised letters for the blind) about the senses, and in conversation afterward, I told her she had three. She was much displeased because she had not as many as one of the blind girls whom she considers, not without reason, as decidedly her inferior.* After sitting still a moment this morning, apparently thinking earnestly, she said, " I have four." " Four what?" " Four senses; think, and

---

* When this child entered school Laura took her under her special care, showed her about the house and assisted her in various ways, but in trying to teach her the finger alphabet she discovered her mental incapacity, and afterwards manifested a decided aversion to her. If anything were broken or lost, she always attributed it to Olive.

nose, and mouth, and fingers. I *have* four senses."
And she seemed much delighted at the discovery.

June 16. Laura began to learn the multiplication-
table. Found she knew the two table perfectly, though
after reciting it she said, " My think is very tired."

She corrected me for not saying " please " in every
sentence. She had some cake given her, and said she
must give Lucy some, but first wished me to teach her
to spell it with the types. Told Laura it was " pound "
cake, and laughing she pounded upon her desk. This
is the only meaning she has yet been taught of that
word.

June 18. As an exercise upon the two and three
tables, gave her to-day an example on the board. This
pleased her much, and she worked with great spirit.
While walking on the piazza, she said, " Why do sun
not come?" Because clouds are over it. " Who shut
clouds? "

June 19. One of the gentlemen who visited the
school to-day saw Laura when she first came to the
Institution, and desired to know if she would recognize
him by touching again his finger-nail, which was of a
peculiar shape. She touched his hand, perceived the
nail, and turning to one of the blind girls who stood
near, said, " I remember to see man when it was very
cold. I could not talk with fingers. I did not know
(then) man had got any name."

Heard a sound from both Lucy and Laura this morning that led me to think all was not right. Found that
Laura had accidentally broken the string of Lucy's fan
while playing with her, and that Lucy was taking re-
venge by pinching and striking, while Laura, not under-

standing about it, still kept her arm round Lucy. This
made matters worse; and she had worked herself into
quite a passion before I got to her. Separated them,
and Lucy grew calm, but Laura was much troubled.

On coming for her lesson Monday morning, she said,
" I want to talk much with you." Her first topic
was the trouble with Lucy. She had been thinking
about it, and could not understand it. " Why did Lucy
pinch and scratch me? Was she very wrong?" Tried
to excuse it, saying she did not know better. " Did she
know I was very sorry to break her fan? Why will
Lucy pinch and strike?" Told her I hoped she would
soon learn it was wrong, and we must be patient with
her. This being settled to her satisfaction, she said,
" Why do not heart stop?" Being puzzled for a reply
that should not involve me in questions I was not allowed
to answer, I said, " Because it cannot stop." Told her
she always breathed. She held her breath for a while,
and said, " I do not breathe now." But you will breathe
soon, and cannot stop long, or it will hurt you. "And
die," she added. " Is not heart very tired?"

She seems to have a theory of her own regarding
the seat of sensation. During a lesson one day she
stopped, and holding her forehead, said, " I think very
hard. Was I baby, did I think?" (meaning, when I
was a baby). Another day she said, "Doctor will come
in fourteen days, I think in my head." Asked her if
she did not think in her side and heart. " No; I cannot
think in heart; I think in head." Why? "I cannot
know; all little girls cannot know about heart." When
disappointed or troubled, she often says, " My heart
aches." One day she asked, " When heart aches, does

blood run?" We had told her about the circulation of
the blood. "Does blood run in my eyes? I cannot feel
eyes blood run. Why cannot I stop to think? I cannot help to think all days. Do you stop to think?
(meaning, cease thinking). Does Harrison stop to
think, now he is dead?" President Harrison had lately
died, and the blind girls had talked much about it and
by them Laura had been told of it.

June 24. Within the past week Laura has begun to
ask the color of everything. We cannot find where she
got the first idea of it. This morning she would have
liked to devote her whole lesson to it, she was so much
interested. She has attached an idea of inferiority to
red, and was displeased when told a dress, which she
wore in the afternoon, had red in it, and said, " I will
wear it in the morning."

June 25. Continued the subject of color, and her
first question was, "What did man make red for?"
Told her because l·e thought red pretty, and that
reconciled her to it. I tried unsuccessfully to find,
by questioning, the origin of her dislike, but can only
venture a surmise that the article she had in her hand
when first told of the color red, may have been harsh
and disagreeable to her touch.

This leads me to speak of my observations with
regard to the power of the blind to distinguish
color. Fabulous stories have been told, but certainly among the pupils at our Institution, there
were none of whom we could make similar statements. It is true of many totally blind that, if a
number of balls of worsted of various colors are

given them, and they are obliged to notice them carefully, that they may use them in their proper places in work, they will rarely make a mistake. So we may give them pieces of silk, with the same result, but this does not prove, that having been told the colors in one material or fabric, they will recognize them in any other.

We have no evidence that there is any inherent property in the color red, or blue, or yellow, which will enable the most sensitive touch to detect each in all materials offered.

It has often been stated by letter-writers that "Laura Bridgman can tell the color of everything by feeling." This we know is a mistake, and as we suppose her sense of feeling to be more acute than that of any other person, we infer that it cannot be *literally* true in any case.

June 26. Sent Laura to bring Lucy down to the school-room. She came, looking quite sad, and said, "Lucy talked with her mouth." "What did she say?" "I cannot know. Lucy *did* talk." She was comforted by my assuring her she only made noises, it was not talking. She must have had her hand near Lucy's mouth, and perceived some motion similar to talking.

June 28. In the midst of an arithmetic lesson she stopped to ask the name and color of her eyelashes and brows. When talking of hair, she asked the color of mine, and said, "Mine will be dark brown too when I am tall." She walked to the window, where the lower shutter was closed, and said, " I will talk about this,"

and asked the name and color of the hasp and hinge,
then swinging it backward and forward said, "It is like
a clock " (pendulum).

June 29. She brought her doll into school, and said,
" It is not pretty to bring doll into all schools," and
then extended its hand towards me, and said, "See doll
talk," and moved its fingers to spell " Swift." She was
delighted that I could understand it, and said, " Doll
can talk with fingers ; I taught doll to talk with fingers."
She has lately made a strange noise which she calls
" calling," and if I leave her a moment she makes it,
and says, " I wanted you to come and I called you."

This is quite a new idea, as all the noises she
has previously made were evidently not intended to
attract attention. Of these Dr. Howe speaks in
one of his reports as follows : —

" It may be well to explain what was said in a
former report about Laura making a peculiar sound
whenever she meets any person, which she calls that
person's *noise,* and about which many inquiries have
been made, especially as an important physiological
inference may be drawn from it. When she meets me,
one of the pupils, or any intimate friend, she instantly
makes a noise with the vocal organs ; for one a chuckle,
for another a cluck, for a third a nasal sound, for a fourth
a guttural, etc. These are to her evidently signs, or
names affixed to each person. These are known by
those very intimate with her , when they speak to her
of such and such an one, she makes her ' noise " ; and
these noises or names have become so intimately associated with the persons that sometimes, when she is

sitting by herself, and the thought of a friend comes up in her mind, she utters his ' noise,' as she calls it, that is, what is to her his name. Now, as she cannot hear a sound, as she never attempts, like deaf and dumb persons, to attract the attention of others by making a noise, it follows that, impelled by the natural tendency of the human mind to attach signs to every thought, she selects the natural vehicle for the expression of it, and exercises the vocal organs, but without any definite view of producing an effect. This would seem to prove, if indeed any proof be wanting, that men did not select vocal sounds for a colloquial medium, from among other possible media, but that it is the natural one."

July 1. Laura did not succeed as well as usual in her arithmetic, and was a little fretful and impatient. When her examples were corrected, she was quite displeased, and said, "Ladies do not say wrong. I think you are very wrong to say wrong to me. Think cannot do good, because I am very deaf. Think is very long," meaning slow in working.

July 2. A complaint was entered against Laura that she pinched Lucy and made her cry. I talked with her about it, and said to her, " Lurena told doctor you pinched Lucy's nose and made her cry." Before I had finished the sentence she smiled, and seemed, by the expression of her face, to think that it was very ridiculous to pinch her nose ; but when she was told that Lucy cried, she changed countenance, and was immediately sad. She said, " When did I pinch Lucy's nose?" I replied, "Lurena said yesterday." "After how many schools?" I told her I did not know. She thought a moment, and then said eagerly, " I pinched Lucy's nose after one * school, to play. I did not mean to make her cry, because I played. Did Lucy know I was wrong?" I told her Lucy did not know when she played, and she must play softly. I asked her if she loved Lucy; she replied, "Yes, but Lucy does not hug me." "Why does she not?" "Because she is very deaf and blind and does not know how to love me; she is very weak to hug."

July 3. Gave Lucy the word "cake" and called Laura to spell it to her; the interest seemed to be all on Laura's side, as she cares much more than Lucy about the lessons. She asked with great earnestness, "Does Lucy know what I say?" and added, "I want her to learn to talk very, very" (and to make it emphatic, she repeated it ten times) "much."

July 8. Laura went to ride, and as usual asked the color and name of the horse. Told her "Post-boy." She said, "What boy? Has he four legs?" She was puzzled by the name, and could not decide whether it was man or horse.

July 9. Laura was ready for her lesson before prayers, and when I went down, led me to the table to show me a box and asked "What?" It was fastened with hasps, and looked as if it had not been opened, but to satisfy myself of her self-denial I asked her if she had opened it. She said "No" with great emphasis, showing thereby her nice sense of propriety. Allowed her to open it, and she was surprised when told it was for her to use. It contained types with raised letters on the end, and had grooved lines in which they could be set up.

The next morning she brought the box with the

---

* She was accustomed to reckon time by schools, "a school," with a recess of a quarter of an hour, occupying an hour. The first "school" was before breakfast, closing at seven o'clock.

alphabet arranged in order seven times, and the remainder of the types in such a way that she knew where to find them. This had taken her several hours to accomplish, but much gratified her strong love of order.

July 13. This was a sad day to us all. Lucy's parents had sent for her to return to them, and all the care and anxiety she had been to her teachers for the five months was forgotten in the sorrow of seeing her leave us. Had she remained we had no doubt of our future success in teaching her, for the greatest difficulties were overcome, but now she must go back from dawn into night again. Laura could think of nothing but Lucy, when she came for her lesson, as she had just bidden her good by. She was much troubled that Lucy did not return her embraces. She said, "I am very sorry; I cannot work much because I am very sorry that Lucy is going away. Why will not Lucy hug me? Will Doctor cry?" Then she reviewed Lucy's history, and not one circumstance connected with her seemed to have escaped her mind. She said, " Doll will cry; she is very sorry Lucy is gone, and will cry."

A week after Lucy left, Laura was told by Dr. Howe of a blind deaf and dumb boy who would come to the school before long. She had many questions to ask : " Can I talk with him when he has learned much? " This question occurred to her mind, I presume, because in the school the boys occupied one part of the house and the girls another, and so she doubted whether she would be allowed to talk with him. " Will you kiss the

little blind and deaf and dumb boy? Why not?"
"Because it is very wrong to kiss boys" (with a
very imperative air).

July 23. She brought me her new board with a very
good sentence set up in types: " Doctor and Drew and
Swift taught Lucy to learn to talk with her fingers, and
Laurena taught her to read on board, good; when
Laura came with my mother, doctor and Drew taught
me on knife and fork and spoon and mug very good."
She said of her own accord, " Laura is wrong" and sub-
stituted "I" for it. She shows much ingenuity in arranging the spaces between the words; she has not enough
blanks for long sentences, and so takes the smaller letters and turns the blank end up. While Miss Drew
was talking with her she asked, " What is by and by?"
and was told it meant soon. She went to her work, but
came back five minutes after, saying, " To and to is
now." Being asked why she thought so she said,
' Because by and by is soon."

July 27. Laura said this morning, " I do not want
to study to cipher, I want to talk about things. What
.s hour? Doctor said after two hours." After talking
some time she said, "Sunday is two hours; eight weeks
Sunday, peaches will grow." Neither remark was intel-
ligible to me. She attended very quietly to my explanation for some time, and said, "I cannot have some
one to say weeks and hours to me, because I cannot
know" (understand). Told her she could know hour,
and tried to explain it as one school and one recess.
Feared she might think them synonymous in meaning
rather than in time, but after sitting still a long time

5

thinking, she said, " After one school, after recess, is an hour, and a week is after Sunday."

When a subject that is very difficult occupies part of the hour, I turn her attention to something which will be easier, but will teach her some new words, so to-day showed her a ball of wicking, taught her the name and color. and throwing it upon the desk she noticed its elasticity, and said, " Ball jumps "; taught her the word " bound."

Aug. 2. Exercised Laura in examples with five for a multiplier. She did them very rapidly and without much effort. In review gave her one with two for a multiplier, and found she had almost entirely forgotten that table while learning the higher numbers. This surprised me, as she never seems to forget in any other study. When she had finished her lesson she found on her board a row of figures without a multiplier, and playfully put down a cipher and commenced multiplying by it.

Aug. 4. Laura's sentence on her board this morn was, " Osborne went on water, he was very tired to work & he came to see his mother. Cyrus came to see Miss Drew. Miss Davis sent berries to girls to eat them for dinner, good. Olive was very wrong to tell .ie when it was very cold." She seemed quite impatient when I wished her to correct it, but was reconciled when told that the reason I wished her to put it on the board was that, by correcting it, I might teach her to talk as other girls do. The letter s was exhausted before she finished the sentence, and I suggested leaving a blank for it, but instead of doing so, she put z in its place.

It was singular that she should have hit on the letter
which sounded most nearly like s, so I asked why she
did not take o or t. " Because o and t are not good,"
was all the reason I could get.

Aug. 16. The sentence this morning was " I, & J,
& Doctor went in the boat to see Betsy Tuesday, & all
the girls went to ride in the cars to See-konk & they
picked many whortle & blueberries. Mr. Greene gave
me some cake & Mrs. Greene gave me raspberries. I,
& Drew, & Martha, went to see baby." Tried to
explain to her that " I " should come after " Doctor,"
but she was much dissatisfied and said, " Why must I "
(pointing to herself) " come last? I rode *between* Dr. &
Jennette." Her manner of writing See-konk with a
dash, showed the idea she attached to the name. When
we came to the last clause I thought she would correct
it herself and put the " I " last, but she objected and said,
" I sat first, why must I be last? "

Aug. 19. Taking up a pincushion which was in the
form of a fish, she said, " What is it "? When told,
she threw it down quickly as if afraid to handle it, then
taking it up again said, " You must teach me about fish.
Why has it not legs? " Described the fins and their use,
then showed her another pincushion in the form of a
fly. She asked the different colors of the silk, and the
use of the various parts. " Why do flies fly with wings?
Why do they not walk on the floor? Because girls would
walk on them, and hurt them very much? Why do flies
get in water? Can you catch fly to show me legs and
wings? Why does not the silk fly move?" I was
about to answer when she showed me one wing was
partly off, and said, " Fly is dead." Asked her if she

thought it flew before it was off, and she seemed to think it did.

Aug. 20. Laura asked to talk about animals, so excused her from the much less interesting lesson in arithmetic. Her mind is full of the subject now. "Why do not flies and horses go to bed? Why do they eat fast? Are horses cross all days? What does horse do? Is he hurry to go? Do horse know it is wrong to go slow? Would they know that carryall would fall if they went slow and the ground was rough? Why does Abner hold the horse's head when we get in? Why did horse fret?" (Shaking her head up and down.) She had probably perceived the jar of the carriage from this motion of the horse, and some one had shown her what the horse did to cause it. Just then a horse came into the yard; she felt the jar and asked, "Why do horse walk hard on barn floor? I will see horse." Told her I would show her one, meaning a model. "Will horse come into school? Do ladies bring horse into school? I think I am very sorry I said I would see horse."

Aug. 23. I found Laura waiting for me with two pieces of paper, one folded very small, which she said was "hopper," meaning it was about the size of a grasshopper; the other, much larger, was "elephant." She was not satisfied with the name hopper, and changed it to "grass-hopper," then to "hopper-ground." I think she had an idea that if she used grass, it would mean that it was made of grass, and so was puzzled what to call it. Next she asked, "What are flies' names?" Being sure she knew better than to ask such a question, I replied, "Ellen and Laura and Susan." She laughed

heartily, and said, "Flies have no name but bug.
Why do not flies have names like girls and boys? Why
do horses have iron shoes? Do they tie them on with
strings? Why do men hold horse's foot to put on
shoes? I hear horse walk when he kicks off flies,
because they are hard." She often perceives the jar
made by the stamping of the horse in the stable.
"Why do cows not draw?" "Cow's feet are cut in two
parts." Told her she might go out to the stable with me
to see the cow's foot. but she shrunk from it, saying,
"No, she would run and kick me. When horses and
cows are sick, do they go to bed like girls and get well?
Do they go down stairs? Why do cows have horns?"
"To keep bad cows off when they trouble them," was
my answer. "Do bad cows know to go away when
good cow pushes them?" After sitting some time in
thought, she said, "Why do cows have two horns, — to
push two cows?" moving her hands in two directions.

Extended reports of conversations are copied
from journals, that the reader may be enabled the
more fully to realize how many things a child thus
isolated has to learn in this way, which we never
know how other children acquire. Dr. Howe
remarks, —

"her curiosity is insatiable, and by the cheerful toil
and patient labor with which she gleans her scanty har-
vest of knowledge, she reproves those who, having eyes
see not, and having ears hear not."

Aug. 24. Lesson upon weeks and months. She
learned to reckon the number of weeks in three, four,
and five months. Asked her if she had done tea

"You are wrong to say tea; it is milk and wate.."
Walked with her to South Boston Point, and showed
her a boat and oars, but could not persuade her to sit
in it, "Because," as she said, "I am afraid it will move."

When asked the next day why she did not make a
sentence on her board about the oars, she replied,
"Thought was very sleepy not to study much." This
is the first time she has made use of the noun "thought,"
her usual expression being "Think is tired." She asked
what bit her, and was told mosquito. "You were wrong
Monday to say flies had no name; it is mosquito fly."

She shook hands with me and laughing said, "I have
been to see your mother; I went yesterday after dinner,
and I came this morning. She said she was very glad to
see me, and I said, 'How do you do?'" She enjoyed
this little play of imagination as a very good joke.
After tea she asked, "Is it very time?" and explained it
by saying, "Is it late?" evidently thinking her first
form more emphatic.

Aug. 30. She is becoming more and more dissatisfied with her type-setting. It is a very slow process for
her, and with all the pains she can take she does not
succeed in setting up as good sentences as she uses in
talking with her fingers. The corrections displease her,
but we are not ready yet to give up the experiment.
She shows great ingenuity often in making excuses, and
so begging off from it. This morning she was full of
them: "I must make many pitchers" (a kind of purse
made in the shape of a pitcher which she had been
taught to knit of worsted, her orders for them being
often in advance of the supply) "for ladies, and they
will not be done." When this excuse did not avail she

said, "I shall not have you teach me after it is cold because I have learned all." Asked if she thought I knew no more to teach her, but she had no answer, only asked, "Why did doctor have Munger make types?" "To teach you to talk like all the girls." "I can talk good now." I could not blame her much for this little pettishness, for I think girls who could see would find their patience taxed.

Laura has a very keen sense of the ludicrous, and while she is sympathetic when she sees any one is hurt, yet her expressions of sympathy will often be supplemented by a good, hearty laugh. An illustration occurred just at this date. Dr. Howe met with an accident. She said, laughing heartily, "I am very sad because doctor hurt him. I want him to be well very much; he hurt his leg, and walked like a dog." Then she laughed again, and said, "I am very much afraid I shall not see doctor walk on crutches for legs; I want you to ask him if he will walk, and let me see him." Another day she had a great play over the letters of the finger alphabet. The letter which amused her most was t, which is made by putting the thumb between the next two fingers. She put her fingers over her nose, so it would project between them, and said "like t." When I took my paper to make notes of the lesson she put her hand on the pencil, and said, "Do not write about nose and thumb; I do not want doctor to know." She probably thought he would call it silly.

Talking about moths one day, she decided very positively that moths ate all old dresses, and that was what made them wear out.

Sept. 6, 1841. Laura wrote the following letter to her mother without assistance : —

DEAR MY MOTHER:

May I come with Miss Drew to Hanover if I will be very good and not trouble mother? Do she want me (to) come to see her? I will try to be good at Hanover. She must write to Drew. I send love to mother. May I make a pitcher (purse) and chain for her and father in Hanover? I send love to father and my brothers. Will mother be very glad to see me and Drew? Swift sends her love to my mother. Swift and Drew taught me good. I will come in vacation. I am well. I ate with Jennette & Doctor. Man pricked paper; he took my face for mother. I was sick. I can sew and study and write and knit. Drew was sick. Lurena cannot walk because she is lame. I sleep with Drew. I shall bring doll.

LAURA BRIDGMAN.

Sept. 9. Laura said, " I will go home after six Sundays "; and added, after stopping some time to calculate, " that would be forty-two days." I replied, " Yes, six times seven are forty-two." I perceived she had arrived at it by addition, and wished her to take the hint of the better way. After a moment's thought I saw it was not lost upon her, for she said, " Yes, like seven." Explained it further, and then asked if she knew now why it was " like seven." " Yes," hesitatingly. " Get beans." After counting them off she was entirely satisfied, and much pleased with her new knowledge.

Sept. 12. Dr. Howe told her a story, which was designed as a test of her conscientiousness. We copy his account of it: "A little boy went to see a lady, and the lady gave him two birds, one for himself and one for his sister; she put them in a basket for him to carry home, and told him not to open the basket until he got home; the boy went into the street and met another little boy, who said, ' Open the basket, and let me feel the birds '; and the boy said, ' No, no '; but the other boy said, ' Yes, yes '; and then the boy opened the basket and they felt of the birds. Did he do right? She paused, and said, ' Yes.' I said, ' Why? ' She replied, ' He did not remember.' I said, ' If he did remember, did he do right? ' She replied, ' Little wrong to forget.' I then went on to say, ' When the boys did feel of the birds one bird was killed.' Here she became very much excited, and manifested the greatest anxiety and distress, saying. ' Why did boy feel hard? Why did bird not fly? ' I went on. ' He carried the basket and birds home, and gave the dead bird to his sister. Did he do right or wrong? ' She said, ' Wrong.' ' Why? ' ' To kill bird.' I said, ' But who must have the live bird, the boy or the girl? ' She said, ' Girl.' ' Why? ' ' Because boy was careless, and girl was not careless.' She was at first a little confused about the persons, but decided promptly the question of right or wrong, both in respect to opening the basket and about who ought to possess the bird.

" She supposed it was all reality, and I could not well

make her conceive the object of the fable. Her mind was for some time entirely occupied with this story, and she afterwards asked, 'Did man knock (strike) boy because he killed bird?' I said, 'No, the boy's heart did knock him. Does your heart knock you when you do wrong?' She inquired about the beating of the heart, and said, ' My heart did knock little when I did do wrong.'

"She asked, 'Why blood came in face?' I said, 'When wrong is done.' She paused and said, 'Blood did come in Olive's face when she did tell lie. Do blood come in your face when you do wrong?'"

Sept. 13. Laura was full of questions about the story which was told her last evening, and which has interested her very much. "How tall were the little boys? Why did he tell lie, and why did he not mind lady? Why did not boy tell true and he was wrong?" Gave her the word "story." "Why did boys and ladies write in book?" Told her boys did not write; they told man the story, and he wrote it. "All leaves?" "Did blood come into his face when he did wrong?" Told her it came into hers when she was wrong. "I am sorry," she added. "It makes your face look red" "And pretty?" That her face should not look pretty when she had done wrong troubled her much. She said, "I feel very bad because boy told lie to make the blood come in his face."

Sept. 16. She gave me an account of killing a mouse last night, and by the aid of a few questions, made out quite a graphic description. "I slept in blind Sarah's room last night, and I was very afraid because mouse came ; I walked on it, and stamped very hard." "How did you know it was a mouse?" "Because I felt hair and tail. I held mouse up, and I was very afraid because he moved and jumped much. He opened mouth and made much noise. I stamped on him and he was very dead and could not move." This seemed a very improbable story, and at first I thought her imagination had been at work, but on going to the room, found the mouse was there, and " very dead," as she said.

In the above account she says, " He made much noise." In talking of the circulation of the blood she insisted that it made a noise, and put my hand on her neck to feel the pulsations, saying, "Sit very still and see if you do not hear it." At another time she was having a lesson about an india-rubber cord and said, "It makes noise when I pull it." Told her I could not hear it, but she was so sure of it that she held it close to my ear, when, to my surprise, I could hear distinctly the motion of the rubber. The only inference which I can draw from all these cases is, that in consequence of the extreme sensitiveness of her touch, she distinguishes the vibrations which we hear, and which she has observed me speak of as sound, or in her vocabulary as " noise," and so whenever she perceives vibrations, she supposes we can hear them. In the last instance her sense of touch was capable of detecting " noise " more quickly than my ear.

Sept. 17. " Do horses draw good when they are

small like me?" " No." " When they are large like
doctor? Why do horses love to have men pat them?
Do horses think? When I went to get water, dog came
to the door." " Was he glad to see you?" " I did
not ask him because he is very dull, because he cannot
talk with his fingers." " Can he talk with his mouth?"
" No." " What does the dog do with mouth?" She
made a noise, as she supposed, like barking. " Do
horses bark? Do dogs bark to ask men for meat for
them to eat, and when they are cross, and when they
are afraid? Do men talk to dogs when they are cross?"
" Yes, they say, 'Be still!'" " With mouth?" She
was quite indignant that dogs should hear when men
spoke with their mouths, and she could not. " Do men
bark? Do mouse bark?"

As an illustration of the difficulties we met in
making her understand accurately words signify-
ing mental operations, we copy the following:—

Sept. 21. Found she had the idea that to punish and
to blame were synonymous, and tried in various ways
to correct it. I said, " Miss Drew blames you when she
thinks you are wrong and tells you so ; blame is to
think you do wrong." She would not wait for me to
explain it further but said, " I was cross when Anna
was here and Miss Drew blamed me." " She blamed
you because you did what you knew was wrong."
" Why did you not say blame to me before?" " Because
we thought you could not know it before." Had we
stopped here, we should have thought she fully understood the word, but she wished to use it more, and said,
" Do Abner blame horses to ride very quick?" " No."

But she insisted that he did, and to illustrate it made the motion of whipping the horse and saying, " Whip." " Horse blames flies." My answer was, " Blame is not to scold, or to whip, or to strike, or to make you sit still and stay in your room ; it is to think you are wrong. I blame you when I think you are wrong. When you are impatient and push me in school, I think you are wrong and I blame you." She listened unwillingly to this explanation, for it was a little too personal to suit. On such occasions, she shows much adroitness in changing the conversation. Now she said, " Do Abner blame to strike pigs?" " Why do hail break grapes?" She was evidently thinking whether the hail was to blame. I replied, " Pigs and horses cannot know when they do wrong, but you and I know, and if we do wrong men will blame us because we know." She said, " Boy came to take grapes, he was very wrong," showing great indignation: " bird came to eat them, and he could not know, because he was very dull," and here she laughed heartily. "Do you blame the bird?" I asked. " No." " Do you blame the boy?" " Yes. I blamed the boy I saw in Laurena's room, because he played very hard," and she made the sign of striking. I said, "I think you *punished* him if you struck him." Told her a story of a little girl who was sent to carry some apples, and then told the lady she did not know about them, and of a dog who came to take meat because he was hungry. The first excited her indignation so much that to a stranger she would have appeared as if in a passion. Asked her, " Do you blame the girl?" "Yes," very emphatically. " Was the dog wrong?" " Yes — no," alternately. I said, " I do not blame the dog,

because he cannot know. I do not blame babies."
She answered this by saying, "Thomas strikes." Told
her, "He is a little boy and knows, so I blamed him,
but Joseph is a baby, he cannot know, because he is not
old enough to think."

Sept. 23. Laura told me this morning doctor said,
"Chair is thing," and laughed as if she thought it quite
absurd. Took the word for her lesson, and she soon
answered correctly when I gave her objects. Then she
asked if well and white were things. Once when she
mentioned an adjective, I inadvertently said, "Yes,"
and she immediately said, "Very wrong." She asked,
"Why do not doctor whip me with stick when I am very
wrong? Men whip horses with sticks." Told her
because we could tell little girls that we blame them
and that it makes us sorry if they do wrong.

A lady visiting the school asked her to write the
words, "Do good and be good," but nothing could
induce her to do it until she had the promise of an
explanation, as she seemed to think it not a proper
sentence to write.

Sept. 28. In speaking of some one who she thought
had not done rightly, she said, "I think she is to blame
very much," proving that the long lesson was understood.

She was told that a little girl had chicken-pox, and
asked, "Why did she eat so much chicken to make her
sick?"

During this month she had frequent sittings for Miss
Peabody, who was modelling a bust. She rather enjoyed
them as times when she could frolic as much as she
liked.

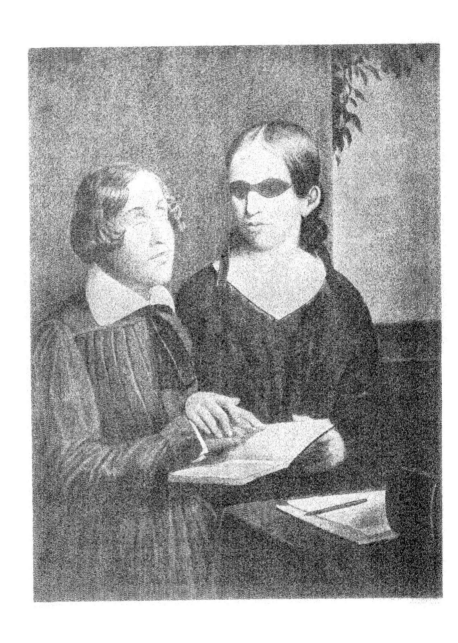

OLIVER CASWELL AND LAURA D. BRIDGMAN, 1844.

Sept. 30. This was a day of great interest both to Laura and myself. Oliver Caswell, the deaf, dumb, and blind boy arrived, and at noon I had the privilege of giving him his first idea of the finger alphabet.* He appeared much delighted with Laura's mode of talking, and imitated her by putting his hand in ours, and making movements with his fingers. He evidently discovered at once that she was like himself, for when he wished to show her anything, he put it in her hand, while he held it up for us to see.

Oct. 1. Dr. Howe gave Oliver a lesson, and he learned to spell many words, and to distinguish between doctor and Swift, when spelled to him. He showed his delight in being taught by laughing heartily after each word in which he was successful. Laura was a most interested spectator, or rather participant, in this lesson, for on the day before, I had not thought best to allow her to be in the room, fearing she would distract his attention. She became so much excited that she forgot herself, and kissed him, and when she came to me for her lesson in the afternoon she was much troubled, and could not speak of it without blushing very much. Yet she seemed to have a conflict in her own mind about it, for she said she thought it was as well as for little Maria to kiss Doctor before she went to bed. After a long talk, she concluded it would be very wrong, '' Doctor would say I was very wrong and would point at me." Evidently her love of appprobation helped her natural modesty in settling the question, and it was a final decision, for I think she never kissed him again.

----

* See Appendix.

Oct. 4. She was surprised this morn to learn that the air was everywhere. She happened to ask me where the wind was to make the fire in the furnace, and explained what she meant by saying, " Match must have air to make it burn, and how could air be in the furnace?" A lesson on trades followed ; she said, " Gown-maker is carpenter, because cloth is made in loom, and man makes cloth." She could not see why a carpenter might not as well do a great many other things, make walls as well as floors.

Oct. 5. She enjoyed her lesson so much yesterday that she came with many questions this morning. Laura gains in one way upon children who have all their senses. If interested in anything specially, she does not forget it, but while dressing, or working, or however occupied, her mind is upon it, while other children go from their lessons into a world which presents so much to take their attention that the lesson is hardly thought of before another school-day comes. To-day she had a long list of things, and wished to know the names of the makers. Was much interested in sailors. The idea that they were sailing day after day, "all days," as she expressed it, was new to her. "Do they go because ladies and men buy things, and men want more to put in store?" Feeling a stone in a ring she asked, " Did mason make rings with stones?" For some time after this lesson she inquired, when introduced to gentlemen, if they were sailors, carpenters, or masons, etc.

One of the greatest trials Laura has is the restraint we are obliged to put upon her in making loud noises. If she is interested in her lessons or excited, pleasantly or unpleasantly, she is inclined to utter sounds which are very disagreeable. She has a pleasant ringing laugh, and we never object to her laughing as much as she likes. She has for a few weeks been trying to be quiet, as Dr. Howe has been away, and she is ambitious to surprise him when he returns.

CHAPTER V.

MISS DREW accompanied her on a visit to her mother in October. They met Dr. Howe in Concord and gave an exhibition of Laura in the State House before many of the citizens.

From this place they went to Hartford, and visited Julia Brace at the Asylum for Deaf-Mutes. When Laura was told she was deaf and blind like herself, she became much excited, and asked, "Can she talk with her fingers?" On being told she had never been taught, she tried to place her fingers in position for the letter a, but Julia's chief interest was in the examination of Laura's dress. The teacher thought that by signs she made her understand they were alike. She also visited Mrs. L. H. Sigourney, who wrote on the occasion the following poem : —

LAURA BRIDGMAN.

THE DEAF, DUMB, AND BLIND GIRL AT THE INSTITUTION FOR
THE BLIND IN BOSTON.

Where is the light that to the eye
Heaven's holy message gave,
Tinging the retina with rays
From sky and earth and wave?

Where is the sound that to the soul
   Mysterious passage wrought,
And strangely made the moving lip
   A harp-string for the thought?

All fled! All lost! Not even the rose
   An odor leaves behind,
That, like a broken reed, might trace
   The tablet of the mind.

That mind! It struggles with its fate,
   The anxious conflict, see.
As if through Bastile bars it sought
   Communion with the free.

Yet still its prison robe it wears
   Without a prisoner's pain,
For happy childhood's beaming sun
   Glows in each bounding vein.

And bless'd Philosophy is near,
   In Christian armor bright,
To scan the subtlest clew that leads
   To intellectual light.

Say, lurks there not some ray of heaven
   Amid thy bosom's night,
Some echo from a better land,
   To make thy smile so bright?

The lonely lamp in Greenland cell,
   Deep 'neath a world of snow,
Doth cheer the loving household group
   Though none beside may know;

And, sweet one, doth our Father's hand
   Place in thy casket dim
A radiant and peculiar lamp,
   To guide thy steps to Him?

At the close of this visit Laura had the grief of
parting with her old and much-loved teacher, who
left her to go to a home of her own. She had
been with her nearly all the time since she came
to the Institution, and to her untiring patience and
perseverance she was indebted for the most of
her early instruction.

Dec. 8. She received an invitation from her old
teacher, Miss Drew, to visit her. This gave her great
pleasure, but she found much fault with her because she
signed her old name Drew, " when her name is Morton
now." Allusion has been made to her habit of making
a different noise for each person : she had one for Miss
Drew, but now she said she must find another, as the
one for Drew must not be the same as for Morton.

Dec. 31. Lesson on Christmas presents, and tried
to interest her in New Year's Day, the number of days
in a year, etc., but she is just now anxious to talk only
on subjects that will furnish new words. " I want you
to tell me new many words. What does language,
syllable, divided, evil, mean ? " She wished me to know
what she had learned, and said, " O ! is when you are
glad, and Oh ! is when we are afraid. Lydia is oh ! of
doctor. Was Lydia naughty and bad to be afraid of
doctor?" It was evident she had been talking with
some of the blind girls and only half understood what
they had tried to teach her.

Having completed the extracts from the journal
for the year 1841, we quote from Dr. Howe's re-

port* a statement of her physical and mental condition at this period : —

" I shall first give an account of what may be called
her physical condition, and its attendant phenomena.
She has had almost uninterrupted health, and has grown
in stature and strength. She is now tall of her age
(twelve years), well proportioned, and very strong and
active. The acuteness of her touch, and of the sense
of feeling generally, has increased sensibly during the
last year. She can perceive when any one touches a
piano in the same room with her; she says, ' Sound
comes through the floor to my feet, and up to my head.'
She recognizes her friends by the slightest touch of their
hands, or of their dress. For instance, she never fails
to notice when I have changed my coat, though it be
for one of the same cut, color, and cloth; if it is only a
little more or less worn than the usual one, she perceives
it, and asks, ' Why?' It would appear that in these
perceptions she employs not only the sense of touch,
but derives great assistance from what Brown would call
a sixth sense, viz., the sense of muscular resistance.
Aided by both of these, she has acquired surprising
facility in ascertaining the situation and relation of
things around her. Especially is it curious to see how
accurate is her perception of the direction or bearing of
objects from her; for by much practice and observation,
she has attained, to some extent, what the bee and some
other insects have in such perfection by instinct, — the
power of going straight towards a given point, without

---

* Tenth Annual Report of the Trustees of Perkins Institution
and Massachusetts Asylum for the Blind.

any guide or landmark. For instance, when she is told to go from any part of the room to a particular door or window, she goes directly and confidently on, not groping, or feeling the walls; she stops at the right instant, raises her hand in the right direction, and places it upon the door-knob, or whatever point she may have aimed at. Of course it is not supposed that she can exercise this power when she is in a new place, but that she has attained great facility in ascertaining her actual position in regard to external things.

" I am inclined to think that this power is much more common than is usually supposed, and that man has the desire and the capacity of knowing all the relations of *outness* (to use a word of Berkeley), so strongly marked as almost to deserve the name of a primitive faculty. The first impulse on waking in the morning is to ascertain where we are, and although the effort to ascertain it may not be apparent in common cases, yet, let a person be turned round when he is asleep, and see how instantaneously on waking he looks about to ascertain his position; or, if he is lying awake in the dark and his bed should be turned round, see how difficult it would be for him to go to sleep without stretching out his hand to feel the wall, or something by which the desire in question may be gratified. Swing a boy round till he is dizzy, look at a girl stopping giddy from the waltz, or a person who has been playing blind man's buff, and has just raised the handkerchief, and mark how, by holding the head as if to steady it, and eagerly looking around, the first and involuntary effort of each one is to ascertain the relations of *outness*. . . . Who could be easy a moment if he had no notion of

what he was sitting or standing upon, or any perception or idea of being supported and surrounded by
material objects?

" Laura, or any blind child, if taken up in a person's
arms, carried into a strange room and placed in a chair,
could not resist the inclination to stretch out her hands
and ascertain by feeling the relations of space and
objects about her. In walking in the street she en-
deavors to learn all she can of the nature of the
ground she is treading on ; but she gives herself up
generally to her leader, clinging very closely to her.
I have sometimes, in play, or to note the effect, suddenly dropped her hand when she was in a strange place
and started out of her reach, at which she manifested
not fear, but bewilderment and perplexity.

" I have said she measures distances very accurately,
and this she seems to do principally by the aid of what
Brown calls the sixth sense, or muscular contraction,
and perhaps by that faculty to which I have alluded
above, by which we attend to the relations of *outness*.
When we ascend a flight of steps, for instance, we
measure several steps with the eye ; but once having
got the gauge of them we go up without looking, measure the distance which we are to raise the foot, even
to the sixteenth of an inch, by the sense of contraction of the muscles ; and that we measure accurately, is proved when we come to a step that is but
a trifle higher or lower than the rest, in which case we
stumble.

" I have tried to ascertain her mode of estimating
distance, length, etc., by drawing smooth, hard substances through her hand. When a cane, for instance,

is thus drawn through her hand, she says it is long
or short, *somewhat* according as it is moved with more
or less rapidity, that is, according to the *duration
of the impression;* but I am inclined to think she
gets some idea of the rapidity of the motion even of
the smoothest substances, and modifies her judgment
thereby.

" I have tried to excite the dormant senses, or to
create impressions upon the brain, which resemble
sensations, by electricity and galvanism, but with only
partial success. When a galvanic circuit is made by
pressing one piece of metal against the mucous membrane of the nose, and another against the tongue, the
nerves of taste are affected, and she says it is like
medicine.

" The subject of dreaming has been attended to, with
a view of ascertaining whether there is any spontaneous activity of the brain, or any part of it, which
would give her sensations resembling those arising
from the action of light, sound, etc., upon other persons, but as yet without obtaining positive evidence
that there is any. Further inquiry, when she is more
capable of talking on intellectual subjects, may change
this opinion, but now it seems to me that her dreams
are only the spontaneous production of sensations,
similar in kind to those which she experiences while
awake (whether preceded or accompanied by any cere-
bral action cannot be known). She often relates her
dreams, and says, ' I dreamed to talk with a person,'
to walk with one,' etc. If asked whether she talked
with her mouth, she says, ' No,' very emphatically,
' I do not dream to talk with mouth ; I dream to talk

with fingers.' Neither does she ever dream of *seeing*
persons, but only of meeting them in her usual way.
She came to me the other morning with a disturbed
look, and said, ' I cried much in the night, because I
did dream you said good by, to go away over the
water.' In a word, her dreams seem, as ours do, to
be the result of the spontaneous activity of the different
mental faculties, producing sensations similar in kind
to our waking ones, but without order or congruity,
because uncontrolled by the will.

" In the development of her intellectual powers, and
in the acquisition of knowledge, not only of language,
but of external things and their relations, I think she
has made great progress. The principal labor has, of
course, been upon the mere vehicle for thought, —
language; and if, as has been remarked, it is well for
children that they do not know what a task is before
them when they begin to learn language (for their
hearts would sink within them at the thought of forty
thousand unknown signs of unknown things which they
are to learn), how much more strongly does the remark
apply to Laura! They hear these words on every side,
at every moment, and learn them without effort; they
see them in books, and every day scores of them are
recorded in their minds. The mountain of their difficulty vanishes fast, and they finish their labor, thinking, in the innocence of their hearts, that it is only
play; but she, poor thing, in darkness and silence must
attack her mountain, and weigh and measure every
grain of which it is composed; and it is a rebuke to
those who find so many lions in the path of knowledge,
to see how incessantly and devotedly she labors on

from morn till night of every day, and laughs as if her task were the pleasantest thing in the world.

" I mentioned some circumstances in my last report, which made me infer her native modesty, and although such a supposition seems to some unphilosophical, I can only say that careful observation during the past year corroborates the opinion then advanced. Nor have I any difficulty in supposing that there is this innate tendency to purity ; but on the contrary, I think it forms an important and beautiful element of humanity, the natural course of which is towards that state of refinement, in which, while the animal appetites shall work out their own ends, they shall all of them be stripped of their grossness, and clad in garments of purity, contribute to the perfection of a race made in God's own image.

" Laura is still so young, and her physical development is yet so imperfect, she is so childlike in appearance and action, that it is impossible to suppose she has as yet any idea of sex ; nevertheless, no young lady can be more modest and proper in dress and demeanor than she is. It has been suggested that, as her father was obliged, when she was young, to coerce her to many things which she was disinclined to do, she may have conceived a fear of every one in man's dress. But on the other hand, she was much accustomed, from childhood, to the society of a simple, kind-hearted man, who loved her tenderly, and with whom she was perfectly familiar ; it was not, therefore, the dress which affected her.

" I may add, moreover, that from the time she came here, she has never been accustomed to be in company

with any man but myself; and that I have, in view of
the future, very carefully refrained from even those
endearing caresses which are naturally bestowed upon a
child of eight years old, to whom one is tenderly
attached. But this will not account for such facts as
the following. During the last year, she received from
a lady a present of a beautifully dressed doll, with a bed
and bedclothes, and chamber furniture of all kinds.
Never was a child happier than she was; and a long
time passed in examining and admiring the wardrobe
and furniture. The wash-stand was arranged, towels
were folded, the bureau was put in place, the linen was
deposited in the tiny drawers; at last the bed was
nicely made, the pillows smoothed, the top sheet turned
trimly over, and the bed half opened, as if coquettishly
inviting Miss Dolly to come in; but here Laura began
to hesitate, and kept coming to my chair to see if I
was still in the room, and going away again, laughing,
when she found me. At last I went out, and as soon
as she perceived the jar of the shutting door, she commenced undressing the doll, and putting it to bed,
eagerly desiring her teacher (a lady) to admire the operation.

" She, as I said, is not familiarly acquainted with any
man but myself. When she meets with one, she shrinks
back coyly; though if it be a lady, she is familiar, and
will receive and return caresses; nevertheless, she has
no manner of fear or awe of me. She plays with me as
she would with a girl. Hardly a day passes without a
game at romps between us; yet never, even by inadvertence, does she transgress the most scrupulous propriety, and would as instinctively and promptly correct

any derangement of her dress, as a girl of fourteen, trained to the strictest decorum. Perceiving, one day, that I kissed a little girl much younger than herself, she noticed it, and stood thinking a moment, and then asked me gravely, 'Why did you kiss Rebecca?' and some hours after, she asked the same question again."

Dr. Howe closes this report with the following remarks upon her ideas of God, and his plans for her future instruction : —

" During the past year she has shown very great inquisitiveness in relation to the origin of things. She knows that men made houses, furniture, etc., but of her own accord seemed to infer that they did not make themselves or natural objects. She therefore asks, ' Who made dogs, horses, and sheep?' She has got from books, and perhaps from other children, the word God, but has formed no definite idea on the subject. Not long since, when her teacher was explaining the structure of a house, she was puzzled to know ' How the masons piled up bricks before floor was made to stand on?' When this was explained she asked, 'When did masons make Jeannette's parlor, — before all Gods made all folks?'

" I am now occupied in devising various ways of giving her an idea of immaterial power by means of the attraction of magnets, the pushing of vegetation, etc., and intend attempting to convey to her some adequate idea of the great Creator and Ruler of all things. I am fully aware of the immeasurable importance of the subject, and of my own inadequacy ; I am aware, too, that, pursue what course I may, I shall incur more of human censure than of approbation ; but, incited by the warmest affection for the child. and guided by the best exercise of the humble abilities which God has given me, I shall go on in the attempt to give her a faint idea of the power and love of that Being, whose praise she is every day so clearly proclaiming by her glad enjoyment of the existence which he has given to her."

CHAPTER VI.

DURING the year 1842 Laura was taught one hour daily by Miss Rogers (Miss Drew's successor) and two hours by myself.

As in the year preceding, there was little system in the course of instruction. Our aim was to improve her language and add to her general information. A review of the work done leads me to say that she advanced despite all disadvantages.

In the extracts from journals which follow, it should be understood that all remarks which are quoted as her own expressions are unchanged, even in orthography.

It was my custom to have lying before me paper and pencil, and the exact words of all sentences which were of interest were noted at once. It may be a surprise that her spelling was so uniformly correct, but when it is remembered that she never makes use of a word without giving its component letters, this is easily accounted for. She has only two ways of using language; the one requires her to make each letter with the fingers, the other to write it with her pencil. She is not led into error by the sound of the word, as children who can hear constantly are, nor by the recollection of its appearance when written; but it is a matter of simple memory, and if that fail, there can be no possibility of spelling by analogy, or in any way making good the deficiency. It becomes a lost word, until such time as it shall be used by some one in conversation with her, and so recovered.

At this time she had only one book which she attempted to read, there being no elementary books printed in the raised type. This was called "The Child's First Book," and while it was all that was required for the blind children, who did not enter the school until they understood ordinary language, it proved a labyrinth of difficulties to Laura, and even at this date a few lines furnished work for a day's explanation.

Jan. 8, 1842. Laura has had a present of a toy range which has a lamp to serve instead of fire She spent the most of her lesson time in asking "the why" of every part, even to the little air-holes in the top of the lamp; nothing escaped her observation. Having satisfied herself on this, she said she had new words which she had found in her book, and wanted me to tell her about, "articulate sounds, vowels, consonants, etc." One would suppose that it would have taken her hours to remember how to spell such words, and the work of explaining them looked equally laborious. The first she soon understood, but I told her no little girls learned about vowels; she must wait till she was older. She replied, " You told me when Miss Drew was here," and then she repeated them, and asked, " What is w and y ? " I supposed she would not be satisfied without an answer to the question why they were called vowels, but as the lesson was continued while taking a walk, she changed the subject. We found four boats drawn up on the shore, which she was very happy in examining; her questions were so numerous it took long to answer them. She had been shown a fish-hook, and supposed that men had to get out of the boats to get the fish in; wanted to know why boats should not have wheels instead of keels. Asked if fire made these boats go. On being told no, she said I was very wrong, that fire was in a large boat. Explained the difference in boats and the use of oars. " Do water roll much and come over men in boat? Who put fishes in water? "

Jan. 13. Laura had found a notice of a Trustees' meeting, which was printed in raised letters, and brought it for explanation. " What are Trustees? " When told they were men who took care of this house, "And the girls and boys? " she added, " and horses? " After a long explanation of " Sir," " Yours respectfully, etc.," I asked her if she knew about it now. " Little, — because you said long words." It always makes her unhappy to be left with a subject half understood, so I went over it all again and explained it to her satisfaction.

Jan. 15. Some one had given her an almanac, and she brought it to me with a sad face, saying, " Jenny sent me book and I cannot know, there are many

hard words on all leaves that I cannot know." Told
her we would talk about it, and I could tell her a great
deal that was in it. So we turned leaf after leaf, and
she wished to be told "everything" there was on a
page, and to have the pictures at the head of each month
explained. The blank leaves for memoranda pleased
her. At the end of the lesson she was as "triumphant
as one who has taken a city," and her comment upon
the one who had told her she could not understand
about it was, "She is very blind, she did not see to
tell me about many things."

It was the wish of Dr. Howe to give her all
ideas concerning death himself, but she often surprised her teachers by use of expressions which had
never been taught her by them. It must be remembered that she was constantly meeting the blind
girls, while passing to and from the school-room,
and she never missed an opportunity for conversation, often holding them unwilling listeners. She
rarely told us of new words or ideas acquired in
this way, at once, but only as they were suggested
to her mind in some lesson. For example, speak-
ng of Cambridge to-day suggested an occurrence
of over a year ago, when she had been at the
Institution only about two years. There were two
little sisters from that place, who were in our
blind family, Adeline and Elizabeth. Adeline
died at her home. She asked, "Did you see
Adeline in box?" "Yes." "She was very cold
and not smooth; ground made ner rough." I

tried to change the subject here, but it was in vain; she wished to know how long the box was, etc., and said, "Drew told me about Adeline : did she feel? Did Elizabeth cry and feel sick? I did not cry, because I did not think much about it." She drew her hands in with a shudder, and I asked if she was cold. She said, "I thought about I was afraid to feel of dead man before I came here, when I was very little girl with my mother; I felt of dead head's eyes and nose; I thought it was man's; I did not know."

I desire to call particular attention to this conversation, and to have the reader distinctly understand the circumstances. A blind, deaf, and dumb child, not over six years old, was led beside a coffin, and her hand placed on the features of a corpse. No one could communicate with her in any way to tell her the meaning of it, and all she could know was the coldness and rigidity, which to her sensitive touch must have been so terrible. Are we surprised that now, when language has been given her, in which she can describe the feelings and tell of the thoughts which must have been indelibly impressed upon her mind, she says she "was afraid," and shudders at the recollecion? She added, "I thought it was man's" (she was correct), "I did not know." Does not this little sentence settle beyond dispute the question, "Can we think without words?"

Jan. 24. She has been thinking much of the lesson on boats and ships, and came to me to ask, if ships were so large and high, how men could get into them. To test her powers of receiving ideas through illustrations that would require her imagination to work quite actively, I built up objects in the room to represent a ship, told her she must think of the floor as being water, and the rug as the ground, and laid a plank to let her see how she could get up to it. She was delighted with it all, and the lesson was a success.

Jan. 29. To-day Laura had the honor of a call from Charles Dickens. His great interest in her caused him to remain for several hours. She was animated in conversation, and I think he received a very correct impression of her.

His "Notes on America" contain several pages of description of this visit.

In this connection I wish to explain, what was perhaps often misunderstood by visitors to Laura, during this period of her life. Out of the fulness of the heart many words of kindness, and many of flattery, were dictated to us to interpret to her. The former we always repeated literally, but we evaded the latter. Persons did not realize that a child placed in her position would naturally become proud, selfish, and disagreeable in many ways, and that more than ordinary care must be taken to guard her from all influences which would produce these effects. When taken to the school-room for exhibition, she was told that the blind

girls were sitting in their desks all around the
room, and that ladies and gentlemen came to see
how the blind could be taught.   She never had an
idea that her share of attention was greater than
theirs, but if the hundredth part of the comments
which were intended to reach her had been repeated, all our efforts to preserve her a modest, simple-hearted child would have been of no
avail.

Feb. 4.   Talking of her plans for vacation, Laura
made an unusually long sentence.   " 1 must go to
Hanover to see my mother, but I shall be very weak to
go far ;   I will go to Halifax, if I can go with you.   If
Dr. is gone away, I think I will go with Jeannette ; * if
Dr. is at home, I cannot go, because he does not like to
be left alone, and if J. is gone he cannot mend his
clothes and fix all things alone."

Feb. 8.   She had written the following letter entirely
without assistance and brought it for me to read.†   It
was directed on the outside to " My Mother, Hanover."

My Dear my Mother :
    I want to see you very much.   I want you to send
me some mince pie, and I want you to write to me.   You
will write letter to me.   I send much love to you, and
Addison, and John (brothers) :   they must send me many
nuts, because I love them very much ;   you must write
to me.   I am very well now, much, my doll is well

---

* Dr. Howe's sister.
† The punctuation marks and capitals are ours.

Lurena is well but she is weak. Miss J. and Dr. are well. Miss Swift and Miss Rogers teaches me many days. Doll is better. I can write with chalk on board. LAURA BRIDGMAN.

Her thoughts were still on her home, and she said, " My mother cried before I came to Boston, because she was very sad to have me come from home. Was she silly? She cannot teach me at home, I should be very dull, and forget all." She then gave me a long description of their rooms, laughed when she told of the low ceilings, little windows, etc., which she compared with those of the Institution.

Feb. 9. Asked if she had any " new words" for me. In reply she said, " Doctor told me about God ; it was very little say, and he told me when I was very tall he would teach me about God much. Is it man? Did it make you and me?" Told her she must ask Doctor again about it.

Feb. 16. Having noticed that Laura was growing careless upon the use of the verbs, devoted the time to a conversation on " do" and " does," which she uses indiscriminately. As an example of the use of " do," she said, " 1 do go to bed " ; and when corrected, asked why it was not as well to omit " go " as " do." She is always ready with illustrations, and after much thinking, was able to correct the sentences herself. She made such mistakes as " I have not been to walk yesterday," " I did not know if she could hear," etc. Asked her if she would try to remember the lesson. " Yes, when I am not in much hurry."

Feb. 17. She brought me a letter she had received,

saying, with great indignation, "Doctor opened and read it to me. Doctor was wrong to open little girl's letters ; little girls open theirself."

Feb. 19. Talked about monkeys. After answering the usual questions which she asks about every new animal, told her a story of one who liked to kiss little girls. Found that she supposed a monkey could talk, and when told he could not, she looked as if much relieved, though she asked immediately if he could see.

Feb. 23. Talking about the veins, told her they were blue ; she asked, " Are they pretty?" This is her favorite color. I drew my finger over them in her neck and face, and it seemed to her very ridiculous that there should be so many colors in her face.

Feb. 25. In the midst of a conversation upon every-day occurrences she said abruptly, " I want to see God. I want Doctor to make me see." Speaking of being tall, asked her if she wished to be tall. " Yes, because I want to learn about many Gods, and to wear collar." It will be perceived that thus far she had only a vague idea of God, but that her desire to be taught about him was very great.

Feb. 28. Laura found a copy of " The Child's Second Book" while left alone on Sunday, and was much pleased that she could understand a sentence here and there. Many words which were new to her she had carefully remembered, and so brought work enough for three or four hours. " Wave, prevent, hollow," she understood readily, and applied the latter to a defective tooth " Cape, point, valleys, plains, and deluge " next occu pied attention. " Drown " was explained " to go under the water, and not come up." " Would they die?"

was her question at once. " Floating, preserved," and lastly " Mediterranean Sea, Bhering's, Narragansett." Told her she would know all about these last when we taught her geography. " Will that be very soon?" Should we not think that a bright child with all her senses had learned a hard lesson if she had committed to memory such a list of words, and then had learned to spell them all correctly? This was just what Laura had done in that hour, when left by herself.

March 5. She wished me to tell her about yarn. Began with the sheep, shearing it, etc. When I got as far as the carding she made the motion for it, and said, " I have seen my mother." Found she was familiar also with the process of spinning. Talked of all the things in the room made of wool. She said, " Silk-worms make something, what is it?" Taught her co-coon, but reserved the story of silk for another lesson. She had been shown a pod with cotton and remembered that the cotton was made from that.

March 7. Yesterday, when reading, she found the word " harmony," and ran to Miss J. and said, " My mother is in book ; it must be Harmony Bridgman, man did not know."

March 9. To show me that she remembered and could apply one of the " new words" of yesterday's lesson she said, on first seeing me this morning, " J.'s hand is instrument to pat with." During the past week she has said several times when checked for making noises, " I thought you could not hear," and instances of this kind have led us to think that she imagined she did nothing wrong, provided she concealed it. To-day taught her the word " deceive," and told her it is to do things when J. is not here that you would not do when she is here. Then gave her several instances of deception which she had used during the last week, all very slight in themselves, but which would fairly come under that head, and thought she began to understand it. She said, "I would not like to have J. know, and I would not like to have Doctor know ; he must make *me* know ; I would be very sad to have any one tell Doctor because he would blame, or scold me." Told her if she did not do wrong no one would have to tell him, and she showed that she fully understood that wrong intent was necessary to make the action wrong by remarking, "I would tell Doctor ; if I did not *mean*, he would not blame me." She has not yet corrected the impression that the error lies in failing to conceal the crime, rather than in its commission. The next day, when sent for her lunch, she found the servant absent, and feeling irritated, took the key from the door to prevent Miss J. from passing through. After talking about it, she said, "I knew it was wrong ; was it deceive?" Told her no, and was about to explain further when she said, "If I do not want J. to know that I took key, it is deceive." Told her that to deceive was a little lie ; that she did not tell large lies, but in this way she could tell many little lies, and it was very, very wrong. She then gave a minute description of the first time she attempted to disobey me, when I was giving her a lesson. Told her I had nearly forgotten all about it, and she said, "You are very forgetful," — the first time I had known her to use this expression.

March 15. Laura was in excellent spirits this morning, for she was expecting Dr. Howe to return after a long absence in the South. She asked, "Do Doctor know I can *smile?*" This is a word she has learned since he went away, and she seemed to think he could not understand it. Among the words she talked of was "fault"; she wanted to know its meaning. Told her it was doing wrong; she said, "Fault is like diameter — no, crime." Accounted for the mistake as I remembered that I taught her both words at the same time and she had crossed their meaning. Explained that fault was a little crime. When walking, she asked, "If the bark of a tree," which I laid her hand upon, "was black, because if it was white it would get dirty?"

March 17. "New words" which she brought to the lesson were, "Mentioned, suit of clothes, approached, arrived." Had her bring me the book in which she had found them, and read a page to me, to see if she got any correct idea of it as a whole. As I supposed, she gave only a confused mixture of words. After reading it, she said, "My head aches to think of many words; do sheep's head ache?" Thoughts of animals, and their points of resemblance to man, seem to be always in her mind. She asked, "Are peaches yellow because they would be dirty if white? and are shoes dark colored?" (for the same reason.) She has lately learned the division of colors into dark and light.

March 26. Laura just recovering from measles. She wanted to know the meaning of "selfish." After a long talk about it, she thought she would like to be a *little* selfish, and I did not succeed in changing her opinion, even by the argument which generally avails much, that ladies do not love selfish girls, and she would not be loved when she grew old if she were selfish.

March 28. Although she was still weak, we had a pleasant talk to-day. Perhaps, as in the case of most people, her sickness has made her think of home and her mother, and she wanted to talk to me of old times. Asked me the names of spindle and reel by describing their motions. She said, "My mother had a swift made of sticks to wind yarn on." She laughed heartily at the name being like mine. She told me about her mother's last visit to her, of the things she brought, and ended by saying, "I think I am *little* afraid of my father." As he had been the one to correct her before she was taught anything, it is not strange she should say this. She speaks of him with affection at other times.

March 30. For several weeks she has had a habit of pushing the blind girls away when she meets them, if she does not wish to speak to them. As it seemed to be growing into a serious matter, both for herself and the blind girls, their esteem for her being somewhat lowered of late, decided to devote an hour to talking about it. When she understood it fully, she was very sad and cried, and felt it very much when I told her the girls would not love her, and why they all loved the gentle Oliver. When it was proposed that she go and tell Abby she was sorry that she pushed her, she went at once, and said, "I shall tell her I am very sad."

April 4. Found Laura much excited over something she had found in a book ; she met me saying, "Doctor wrote in book, 'you must not think because you are blind.'" On referring to it I found she had omitted the conclusion of the sentence, which was, "that you cannot learn as much as other children." I failed to remove the wrong impression entirely, and presume it will still trouble her.

This is one of her greatest difficulties in reading, and it seems almost impossible to teach her how to read properly, *i. e.*, to receive the ideas as a whole instead of detaching sentences, clauses, or even words, and thinking only of their meaning when taken separately, and so failing to get the true sense.

April 6. The experience of the last lesson leads me to think that I cannot better spend an hour with her than in having her read to me from the book with which she has been amusing herself. " I will tell you about the world," was the first sentence, and she stopped to ask, " Who is I ? " Next she read, " It is round," and before reading " like an orange," she told me, " round like a peppermint." The whole of the hour was occupied in making her understand the difference between the shape of the peppermint and the orange.

Dr. Howe came into the room while she was having a lesson, peeling an orange. She stopped in the midst of a sentence to say, " 1 smell orange." We can see a decided improvement in her sense of smell since last year, but she has never noticed any perfume so quickly or at so great a distance before.

April 19. " Why does it rain? " " To make all things grow." " What are all things? " Described the planting of the seed, potatoes, peas, etc., and told her it rained to make them grow, just as she put water on her plant in the pot to make it grow. She led me to it to show me its growth, and found hanging upon it a bunch of raisins, which Miss J. had put there as a surprise. At first she thought the plant had borne fruit, but soon discovered the joke and enjoyed it.

April 21. Lesson on the yardstick; learned to measure three quarters, half, one quarter, and was very happy in applying her new knowledge.

April 25. Another example of her difficulty in reading. The sentence was, "The deer knows this." The previous sentence was, "The grass grows under the snow." She could not put the two together as any other child would readily do, but asked, with a look of great surprise, "Can the deer know what is in this book?"

April 27. When returning from a walk with her, I told her I could see the windows in our house. She asked at once, "Can you see my Hanover's windows?" meaning the windows in her father's house in Hanover, N. H. One day when walking on our piazza, I said, "I can see the windows in the houses in Boston, and the sun shining on them very brightly." Another day when sitting in the room I told her I could look through our window and see the windows in Boston. She said, "Look through their windows and tell me what all folks are doing."

May 2. The dog Marco accompanied us in our walk to-day, and she was much interested in asking the extent of his knowledge. "Can Marco hear when you say Marco?" Told her yes, and that he came to me. 'Does he know Doctor?" "Yes." "Will you say Doctor to him, and see if he knows?" Told her he did not know when I talked about Doctor, but when he saw him he knew him. This was a great puzzle to her, that he should know his own name and not Doctor's, and

after thinking of it for some time she said quite impatiently, " I will ask Doctor, you do not know."

May 3. While walking to the Point two or three
cannon were fired from a vessel near the Farm School.
At each report she said, " I hear; it is cannon."
Thinking she might describe her hearing as she did in
case of the piano, I asked, " Do you hear through your
feet?" " No, when it is very loud I hear in my ear."

May 8. Laura's mind has been entirely occupied
with the sick horse. She wants to know if he has
medicine. "Does he know sick or better?" Told her
he did not know the words, sick or better, but he knew
when he felt better. She asks every hour what they
are doing for him, and if they give him gruel. When
told no, she said I was wrong, that horses ate meal and
water and that was gruel, which I did not dispute. To-
day she had been told he was dead. " Why did not I
die when I was very sick?" This is the first time she
has alluded to her own death in conversation with me,
and now she looked anxious and much troubled. " Did
horse know about dead, before he was dead?" Succeeded in diverting her attention, and she was very
happy for a while. One extreme of feeling is often followed, in her case, by the other. Asked her why she
laughed so much? "Because I am very O." " What
is O?" " When I am very happy: you said ladies say
O. I am very O!" She soon returned to the old subject and said, "I cried much Friday morning because
the horse was worse, and I love him *very* much, he is
soft and gentle."

May 12. Gave her a lesson in the stable; examined
the harness, saddle, bit, blinders, and reins, sleigh-bells,

collar, stirrups. Then took her to the carriage, and
taught her the name of many of its parts, and the use
of the springs.

May 13. Laura had a lesson in multiplication, and
I told her to-morrow I would teach her to divide. She
thought I said " dive " and was quite troubled about it,
but when she found it was divide and something new in
arithmetic, she said, " To-day, not to-morrow."

May 15. Laura asked for " poor pork " at dinner
to-day. Found she wanted lean pork. She often falls
into mistakes in words by false analogies, and it is easy
to see how she should make the above mistake. One
day when feeling ill she said, " I am very strongless."
When corrected she said, " You say restless, when I do
not sit still," and then changed her sentence to, " I am
very weakful."

May 17. Laura succeeded in dividing 252 by 6.
Have commenced teaching her by long division, thinking it less puzzling for her than short. Last night, in my
sleep, I told Laura to go into Miss Jeannette's room.
She obeyed, but this morning severely reprimanded me,
and concluded by saying, " You do not think good in
your sleep."

May 23. I fear that Laura attempted to deceive me
to-day in her work. At ten o'clock I sent her to knit.
She was to commence a pitcher (purse), and I told her
I wanted she should knit much. At twelve I went to
give her a lesson and asked her how much she had
done. She said, " I have done handle and neck," chang
ing it to " and almost neck." Her manner was pecul
iar, so I asked her to let me see it ; she hesitated, but
brought it, when I found instead of the neck being

almost done, it was not yet entirely begun. Told her
I would not give her a lesson again to-day, but she
must think about deceiving. She worked steadily, but
did not seem to be moved by this.

May 24. Her mind was entirely occupied with the
wrong of yesterday. She asked, " Am I wrong many
times?" She then repeated the history of the deception and said, " I felt very bad yesterday, — bad is
sad. I want to learn to be good." Asked if she
thought she would be sad if she learned to be good.
" I do not think so." After thinking awhile, she said,
" I want you to love me many times, much," and burst
into tears. It was some time before she became composed, but after that she was very gentle.

P. M. Walked to the Point, and while sitting by
the water she said, " I was very silly not to think to
wear shawl." After being quiet awhile, she said, " Be
very still, something in my right foot hears." Asked
her to try her left foot. She did so, but said, " I cannot hear good with my left " " What is in right foot
that hears?" Told her the water jarred the ground,
and she felt it shake. " Who put jar under the ground?"
She had seen a jar in the kitchen, so a long explanation
of what I intended for a simple sentence was necessary.

May 27. Laura has been told often that she must
not displace things in the parlor, and yet the figure of a
monk and a little dog belonging to her are always found
turned round and facing the wall. To-day I asked an
explanation, and the reply was, " To have them see the
pictures on the wall."

May 30. Took Laura to see Jane Damon. This
little blind girl had been very singularly afflicted. She

had passed through typhoid fever, but was left by it
with hip-joint disease, and while in the hospital for
treatment, took the small-pox. Of course she had
drawn largely on our sympathies, and Laura had been
greatly interested in her, but had not seen her for
months. She seemed very happy and kissed her, but
in an instant her countenance changed, and she looked
very sad. She had perceived the marks of small-pox
on her face and hands and asked, " What made them?"
Told her Jane had been sick with small-pox. " Not
small-pox," she said earnestly, " it is much pox." Next
she asked her to walk, saying she would help her. She
was very much affected when she found she could not
use her limb at all. A little while after, looking much
distressed, she said, " I am afraid she will die," and
showed me how thin her hair was, and all the marks on
her face. She was comforted somewhat when told
she was nearly well now. Going home, she said, "I
feel very sad, blood does not run, my heart beats very
slow." She then began to devise ways in which we
could all make Jane happy. I never saw Laura so
much affected as when she discovered Jane's condition.

June 11. Told her to-day she must go and *exercise*
in the hall, supposing it would be a new word to her.
As she took no notice of it, I asked her, " What is exercise?" " To run." " Who told you about exercise?"
" No one." " How did you know it was to run?"
" Because you said it would make me well." And then
she tried to spell it, but did not succeed until after several trials. It is the first time I have ever known her
to arrive at the meaning of a word in this way. Having
lost my paper on which I was taking notes, I asked

her to find it. She said, laughing, "I felt it walk away," at the same time taking it from her shoe, and enjoying the joke.

June 14. Gave her another lesson at the sea-shore. The tide had brought in the sea-weed, and it was all new to her. That it should grow on a stone, puzzled her. Next, showed her some with little bags of air, and she applied her new word "elastic" to them, and could feel how hard the sacks were when full of air: then a species with three lobes, which she called fingers. We picked up some that had a little shell attached, and when told there was a fish in it, her questions were numberless. Some of them were, "Why does fish shut in the shell?" meaning, draw himself into it. "Who gave fish shell? Will he live in my hand? Why not from (out of) the water? Is it baby fish?" An hour passed quickly, and then she said, "I think Rogers and Oliver have not seen." So giving me a small stone with sea weed attached, and taking her baby fish, and what she called fingers in her own hand, she went home to teach Oliver.

June 17. She went to get a chair this morning, and finding a large basket with clothes in it, stepped into it. Talked to her some time, to explain the harm she might do to both basket and clean clothes, but she was disposed to excuse herself, saying, "I was blind, and I did not know the basket was there," and changed the subject, saying, "I saw my father's lambs in basket, and a blanket over them, because they would be cold from (out of) basket. Were they wrong to be in basket?" She showed me how her mother placed a chair over the basket, and I told her it was to keep the

8

lambs from jumping out. " Because babies would be
very cold?" Asked her if her mother told her why she
put the chair there. " No; I could not talk to my
mother, and I could not think why she put the chair."
Here was another case of her thinking before she had
any language.

June 21. Laura ran out of the parlor last eve, just
as a gentleman, who was a phrenologist, was examining
her head; when asked why she was so rude, she said
indignantly, ·· Man was not kind to me, and troubled
me, and I did not like to have him put his hand on my
head." She discovered that the fingers of her left hand
were not so pliable as those of the right, and at once
gave the reason, " Left hand never talks."

July 27. Told Laura as I was going with her to the
school-room that a spider was running over my hand,
and had made a web to the floor. This furnished a
subject for the lesson. After describing the process of
spinning the web, told her about its shape, and she
turned to her desk to find " The Child's Book," which
has a plate of the Planetary System in raised lines,
thinking from my description of the web that this must
be a picture of one. As usual, she had many questions
about spiders. When told they ate flies, she asked,
·· Do large spiders eat ten flies? Do they eat them to
keep them from getting into molasses?"

July 28. Laura met me to-day with, " I am very
neat"; and as she had on a clean dress, it was a good
application of a new word. Then she put out her foot,
and asked, " What do ladies wear on their feet?" which
was a delicate way of attracting my attention to some
new shoes.

Aug. 1. Laura was disobedient to Miss J. this morning, in leaving her room to go to the school-room, after having been told not to go out. She thought it a sufficient excuse that she wanted to go to ask Miss W. to tell her about clams. As there had been several cases of slight errors in this way, I made it a subject for conversation, and afterwards asked her if she had done right. She said, " No, I did not obey J." It usually takes a very short time for her to see the error.

Aug. 19. She asked where I would go in vacation, and when told to Nantucket, she tried several times to spell it, and said, " It is very hard." I cannot understand why she always finds so much difficulty with this name, for she learns those which appear to me much more difficult, such as Philadelphia, with very slight effort, while every time Nantucket occurs, she has to learn to spell it anew.

CHAPTER VII.

ONE of the blind boys died, and we give Dr. Howe's account * of his conversation with Laura ·

" One of our pupils died, after a severe illness, which caused much anxiety in our household. Laura, of course, knew of it, and her inquiries after him were as frequent and as correct as those of any one. After his death I proceeded to break it to her. I asked her if she knew that little Orrin was very sick. She said, 'Yes.' 'He was very ill yesterday forenoon,' said I, 'and I knew he could not live long.' At this she looked much distressed, and seemed to ponder upon it deeply. I paused awhile, and then told her that 'Orrin died last night.' At the word *died* she seemed to shrink within herself, there was a contraction of the hands, a half-spasm, and her countenance indicated not exactly grief, but rather pain and amazement, her lips quivered, and then she seemed about to cry, but restrained her tears. She had known something of death before, she had lost friends, and she knew about dead animals, but this was the only case which had occurred in the house. She asked about death, and I said, ' When you are asleep does your body feel?' 'No, if I am very asleep.'

* Eleventh Report to the Trustees.

'Why?' 'I do not know.' I tried to explain, and used the word *soul.* She said, ' What is soul?' ' That which thinks, and feels, and hopes, and loves,' said I, to which she added interrogatively, 'And aches?' Here I was perplexed at the threshold by her inquiring spirit, seizing upon and confounding material and immaterial processes. I tried to explain to her that any injury of the body was perceived by the soul; but I was clearly beyond her depth, although she was all eagerness to go on. I think I made her comprehend the difference between material and spiritual operations. After a while, she asked, 'Where is Orrin's think?' ' It has left his body and gone away.' ' Where?' 'To God in heaven.' 'Where, up?' (pointing up.) 'Yes.' ' Will it come back?' 'No.' ' Why?' said she. ' Because his body was very sick and died, and soul cannot stay in a dead body. After a minute she said, ' Is breath dead? Is blood dead? Your horse died, where is his soul?' I was obliged to give the very unsatisfactory answer, that animals have no souls. She said, ' Cat does kill a mouse, why? has she got soul?' *Answer:* 'Animals do not know about souls, they do not think like us.' At this moment a fly alighted upon her hand, and she said, ' Have flies souls?' I said, 'No.' ' Why did not God give them souls?' Alas for the poverty of her language! I could hardly make her understand how much of life and happiness God bestows even upon a little fly.

"Soon she said, 'Can God see, has he eyes?' I replied by asking her, ' Can you see your mother in Hanover?' 'No.' 'But,' said I, 'you can see her ⌒ ⌐ your mind, you can think about her, and love her. 'Yes,' said she. 'So,' replied I, 'God can see you and all people and know all they do, and He thinks about them, and loves them, and He will love you and all people if they are gentle and kind and good, and love one another.' 'Can He be angry?' said she. 'No, He can be sorry, because he loves all folks, and grieves when they do wrong.' 'Can He cry?' said she. 'No. The body cries because the soul is sad, but God has no body.' I then tried to make her think of her spiritual existence as separate from her bodily one; but she seemed to dislike to do so, and said eagerly, 'I shall not die.' Some would have said she referred to her soul, but she did not; she was shrinking at the thought of physical death, and I turned the conversation. I could not have the heart to give the poor child the baneful knowledge before I had prepared the antidote. It seems to me that she needs not the fear of death to keep her in the path of goodness."

After reporting this conversation Dr. Howe adds : —

"It would have been exceedingly gratifying to be able to announce a more perfect development of those moral qualities on which true religion is founded ; but it was hardly to have been expected ; those qualities are among the last to develop themselves, and are of tardy growth ; we could have *forced* them out perhaps by artificial culture but that would have been to have obtained a hot-house plant instead of the simple and natural one that is every day putting forth new beauties to our sight. It is but thirteen years since Laura was born ; she has hardly *lived* half that number, yet in that time what an important mission has she fulfilled ! How much has she done for herself, how much has she taught others ! Deprived of most of the varied stimuli furnished by the senses, and fed by the scantiest crumbs of knowledge, her soul has nevertheless put forth the buds of the brightest virtues, and gives indication of its pure origin and its high destination."

Having given Dr. Howe's account, and his views of her present mental condition, I quote from my journal a report of conversations with different members of the family : —

When I returned from church found Laura in a very excited state, and as no notes had been taken of her conversation with Miss J. and Miss Rogers, I collected it from them, and also noted that with myself. She came up from the Doctor's room saying, "Orrin has gone to God. Soul has gone. God gives all folks, and men, and boys, and babies, souls. God is very kind." She spoke of the body, and Miss Rogers asked her why she did not say Orrin. "Because Orrin has gone to God." When she met me in the afternoon, she said, "Did you know Orrin was dead? Are you glad?" Turning to Miss J. "Do God love Orrin? Can Orrin move with God?" Then drawing back a little, "I want to be with God. God is very good to give us all souls. God would be sad Orrin's body is dead. Does God know all names and things?" "Yes, and Doctor knows all things God would think that Orrin's soul came from body, — so il came very quick from body

last night. Why did he die? Why did soul go very
quick? Was he any well with God last night?" Her
idea in this question evidently was, whether the soul,
having just left the sick body, began to be well with
God. " Can he talk? Doctor knows about heaven; I
shall know all things when I die." She then made a sign
of drawing out something from herself which was very
thin, and would pass through her fingers, and said,
" Souls are white. Can baby know God? I think I
was with God in Hanover, and God made new Laura."
This was an allusion to her birth. " My doll can see
body, but not soul. Flies and hoppers have not souls.
Shall I go up when I die? Where is God? Are clouds
in heaven?" During the week she often recurred to the
conversation with Doctor, and was much impressed with
the thought, " God knows my thoughts, and wrong, and
does not love bad." One day she said, " Do you want
to see Orrin? Why does not God take us? Does he not
want you and me? Why did God kill Orrin?"

Nov. 15. Laura met a very old lady, and asked,
when she took her hand, " Why did God make her skin
ugly?"

Nov. 16. Walked with Laura. She wore a bonnet
which Miss J. had given her, and said, " I think she is
very kind. What could I do if I had no friends to give
me things?" To deepen this impression, told her a
story of a poor little girl who had no father or mother,
and no home to live in, and who slept in barns. She
was much interested and deeply moved by it.

Dec. 19. For several months I have been unable,
from pressure of other duties, to devote much time to
Laura, but to-day have returned to the pleasant work,

Asked her why she did not read now in her book. " I never read now, I do not know what the words mean." Proposed her reading to me, but she asked that she might tell me about an elephant. Told her a story of little boy who troubled one, and how he retaliated. I chanced to say *he thought.* She did not interrupt the story, but at its close said, " Can elephants think?"

Dec. 21, 1842. Laura announced her birthday. " I am thirteen now : am I taller? "

A very good gymnasium had been fitted up for the use of the blind pupils, and it was thought best for Laura to join the girls at their hour. She was not much pleased with it. As she could not hear the orders and make the movements in concert as those only blind could, it was not strange that some of the charm of it was lost on her.

She visited a museum yesterday, and I asked her to tell me what she saw. " I saw crocodile and elephant's bone of head ; why was his eye very large? I saw elephant's trunk and camel's legs ; they were very high. I could not reach his head, and I stood on stool, and could not reach. Why cannot he put his head to the ground? I saw bear ; what does he do? " After thinking awhile she said, " Why did God make proboscis, and why does the elephant not have teeth and lips like us? "

She wanted to have me tell her about the cages in which bears were kept. After paying close attention, she said, " I will get something to show you if it is like." She went to the apparatus case, and took the little carriage from the inclined plane, to illustrate her idea of a cage on wheels. To give her a more correct one I took the wire frame used with the air pump, and put that on wheels. She understood it at once, but asked, " Why do not bears have cages made of wood? " " They could not have air enough to breathe." She then tried to see if she could feel the air passing through ,he wire. " I sit in my closet many days, and I can breathe, and that is wood." " But you could not breathe if shut up in your desk " ; and this she accepted. As her mind develops she is more inclined to argue, and will not accept an assertion as readily. She told me that bears had glass eyes, and insisted upon it. " I saw dead bear's glass eyes yesterday."

Before closing the account of the progress made for the year 1842, we quote again from the report of Dr. Howe : —*

" Her health has been excellent during the year, un-interrupted, indeed, by a single day's illness. Several medical gentlemen have expressed their fears that the continual mental excitement which she manifests, and the restless activity of her mind, must affect her health, and perhaps endanger the soundness of her mental faculties ; but any such tendency has been effectually counteracted by causing her to practise calisthenic exercises, and to take long walks daily in the open air, which on some days extend to six miles. Besides, she has a safeguard in the nature of her emotions,

---

* **Eleventh Annual Report to Trustees.**

which are always joyful, always pleasant and hopeful; and there is no doubt that the glad flow of spirits which she constantly enjoys contributes not only to her physical health, but to the development of her mind.

" Laura generally appears, by the quickness of her motives and the eagerness of her gestures, to be in a state of mind which in another would be called unnatural excitement. Her spirit, apparently impatient of its narrow bounds, is, as it were, continually pressing against the bars of its cage, and struggling, if not to escape, at least to obtain more of the sights and sounds of the outer world. The signs by which she expresses her ideas are slow and tedious; her thoughts outstrip their tardy vehicle, and fly forward to the goal; she evidently feels desirous of talking faster than she can, and she loves best to converse with those who can interpret the motion of her fingers when they are so rapid as to be unintelligible to a common eye. But with all this activity of the mental machinery, there is none of the wear and tear produced by the grit of discontent; everything is made smooth by the oil of gladness. She rises uncalled at an early hour; she begins the day as merrily as the lark; she is laughing as she attires herself and braids her hair, and comes dancing out of her chamber as though every morn were that of a gala day; a smile and a sign of recognition greet every one she meets; kisses and caresses are bestowed upon her friends and her teachers; she goes to her lesson, but knows not the word *task;* she gayly assists others in what they call housework, but which she deems play; she is delighted with society, and clings to others as though she would grow to them; yet she is happy when sitting alone, and smiles and laughs as the varying current of pleasant thoughts passes through her mind ; and when she walks out into the field she greets her mother Nature, whose smiles she cannot see, whose music she cannot hear, with a joyful heart and a glad countenance ; in a word, her whole life is like a hymn of gratitude and thanksgiving.

" I know that this may be deemed extravagant, and by some considered as the partial description of a fond friend, but it is not so ; and fortunately for others, particularly because this lesson of contentment should not be lost upon the repining and ungrateful, she is a lamp set upon a hill whose light cannot be hid. She is seen and known of many, and those who know her best will testify most warmly in her favor.

" The general course of instruction pursued during the past year, corresponding as it does with that detailed in former reports, needs not to be here repeated for the information of those to whom this report is immediately addressed ; but as great public interest is excited in this case, and as inquiries are continually made respecting the processes by which instruction is conveyed to her mind, it may be well to explain some of them, even at the risk of repetition, and of saying what may seem to those familiar with the theory of teaching the deaf and dumb not only trite but worthless.

" Some kind of language seems necessary for every human being ; the cravings of the social nature are loud and constant, and cannot be gratified except by some medium of communication for the feelings. The ntellect cannot be developed unless all the modifications of thought have some sign even by which they can be recalled. Hence men are compelled by a kind of inward force to form languages ; and they do form them under all and every circumstance. The social organ presents the natural and most perfect medium through which, by attaching a meaning to every modulation of voice, a perfect system of communication is kept up. The question whether a people could exist without language, would be about as reasonable as it would be to ask whether they could exist without hands ; it is as natural for men to converse as it is for them to eat ; if they cannot speak, they will converse by signs, as, if they had no hands, they would feed themselves with their toes. Children then, prompted by nature, associate their thoughts with audible words, and learn language without any special instructions. If you make the sound, represented by the letters a-p-p-l-e, when you hold up the fruit to a child, he naturally associates that sound with it, and will imitate the sound, even without your trying to make him do so ; if the child be deaf so that ie cannot hear the word which you speak, of course he cannot imitate it, and as such, of course, he must be forever dumb But the desire to associate the thing with a sign still remains, and he has the same power of imitation as others, except in regard to words ; if, therefore, you make a visible sign when you show him the apple, as by doubling the fist, the fist afterwards becomes to him the name or sign for the apple. But suppose the child cannot see the apple, suppose he be blind as well as deaf. What then? He has the same intellectual nature. Put the apple in his hand, let him ꞌeel it, smell it, taste it ; put your clinched hand in his at the same time, and several times, until he associates this sign with the thing, and when he wishes for the fruit he will hold up his little fist and delight your heart by this sign, which is just as much a word as though he had said ' apple ' out aloud.

" Reasoning in this way, I undertook the task of instructing Laura Bridgman, and the result has been what it will ever be where nature is followed as our guide.

" This simple process is readily understood ; but simple signs and names of objects being easy enough, it is often asked, How can a knowledge of qualities which have no positive existence be communicated? Just as easily, and just as they are taught to common children ; when a child bites a *sweet* apple or a *sour* one, he perceives the difference of taste ; he hears you use one sound, *sweet*, when you taste the one ; another sound, *sour*, when you taste the other. These sounds are associated in his mind with those qualities. The deaf child sees the pucker of your lips or some grimace when you taste the sour one, and that grimace perhaps, is seized upon by him for a sign or a name for *sour ;* and so with other physical qualities. The deaf, dumb, and blind child cannot hear your sound, cannot see your grimace ; yet he perceives the quality of sweetness, and if you take pains to make some peculiar sign two or three times, when the quality is perceived, he will associate that sign with the quality and have a name for it.

" It will be said that the qualities have no existence, being mere abstractions, and that when we say ' sweet apple ' the child will think it is a compound name for the individual apple, or if he does not do this, that he cannot know whether by the word 'sweet' we mean

the quality of 'sweetness' or the quality of 'soundness.' This is true; at first the child does not know to
what the sound 'sweet' refers; he may misuse it often,
but by imitation, by observation, he at last gets it
right, and applies the word 'sweet' to everything whose
qualities revive the same sensation as the sweet apple
did; he then uses the word 'sweet' in the abstract, not
as a parrot, but understandingly, simply because the
parrot has not the mental organization which fits it to
understand qualities, and the child has. Now the
transition from physical to mental qualities is very easy;
the child has dormant within his bosom every mental
quality that the man has; every emotion and every passion has its natural language, and it is a law of nature
that the exhibition of this natural language calls into
activity the like mental quality in the beholder. The
difference between joy and sorrow, between a smile and
a frown, is just as cognizable by a child as the difference
between a sweet apple and a sour one; and through the
same mental process by which a mute attaches signs to
the physical quality, he may (with a little more pains)
be made to attach them to the moral qualities.

"Much surprise has been expressed by some who are
conversant with the difficulties of the teaching, etc., of
mutes, that Laura should have attained the use of verbs
without more special instruction. It may be said in
reply that no minute and perfect account of the various
steps in the process of her instruction has ever yet been
published; and that moreover the difficulties in the use
of the verbs are in reality much less than is usually
supposed.

"As soon as a child has learned the use of a noun, as

' apple,' and of one or two signs of qualities, as ' sour '
and ' sweet,' he begins to use them, he holds up the
fruit and lisps out, ' apple sour,' or ' apple sweet '; he
has not been taught a verb, and yet he uses one ; he
asserts the one apple to be sweet the other to be sour ;
he in reality says mentally, ' apple is sweet apple,' or
' apple is sour apple ' ; and in a little while he catches by
the ear an audible sign, — the word *is,* — and puts it in
where he before used only a sign, or meant to use one.
Just so with the deaf-mute ; when he has learned a noun
and an adjective he uses them by the help of a verb, or
some mark of assertion, and you have only to give him
some sign, which he will adopt just as readily as the
speaking child, by mere imitation and without any process of ratiocination. We give too narrow a definition
when we say a verb is a word, etc.

" But it would swell the report to a volume should I
pursue the same train of remarks with regard to the
different parts of speech. Indeed I should hardly have
hazarded it here, had it not been for assertions, emanat-
ing from respectable sources, that this child must have
some vision or hearing, or some remembrance of oral
language, since she has easily attained the use of the
most difficult parts of speech, which cost so much labor
to those merely deaf and dumb. It is needless to repeat
what is so well known to hundreds, that she is totally
deaf and blind, and has been so from her tender
infancy.

" It will be observed by those who have had the
patience to read the above remarks that to the child
with all his senses, the acquisition of a language, which
has already been perfected by the labor of many succes-

sive generations, is an easy and pleasant task, and accomplished without any teacher; that for the deaf-mute the difficulty is increased a thousand-fold; that for the deaf, dumb, and blind, it is immeasurably greater still; and that for poor Laura Bridgman it is even more increased by the fact that she has not that acuteness of smell and taste which usually aid those in her situation, and that she relies upon touch alone. Nevertheless, she goes on, joyously using her single small talent, patiently piling up her little heap of knowledge, and rejoicing as much over it as if it were a pyramid."

Dr. Howe's views with regard to her religious training, as given in the same report, are as follows : —

"The various attempts which I have made during the year to lead her thoughts to God and spiritual affairs have been, for the most part, forced upon me by her questions, which I am sure were prompted by expressions dropped carelessly by others, as God, heaven, soul, etc., and about which she would afterwards ask me. Whenever I have deliberately entered upon them, I have done so with caution, and always felt obliged by a sense of duty to the child to make the conversation as short as possible. The most painful part of one's duty is often where an honest conviction forces one to pursue a line of conduct diametrically opposite to that recommended by those for whose superior talents and wisdom one has the greatest respect. It is said continually that this child should be instructed in the doctrines of revealed religion; and some even seem to

imagine her eternal welfare will be perilled by her
remaining in ignorance of religious truths.   I am aware
of the high responsibility of the charge of a soul, and
the mother who bore her can hardly feel a deeper interest in Laura's welfare than I do ; but that very sense of
responsibility to God, and that love I bear to the child,
forces me, after seeking for all light from others, finally
to rely upon my own judgment.   It is not to be doubted
that she could be taught any dogma or creed, and be
made to give as edifying answers as are recorded of
many other wonderful children to questions on spiritual
subjects.   But as I can see no necessary connection
between a moral and religious life and the intellectual
perception of a particular truth, or belief in a particular
creed, I see not why I should anticipate what seems to me
the course of nature in developing the mental powers.
Unaided by any precedent for this case, one can look
only to the book of nature ; and that seems to teach
that we should prepare the soul for loving and worship-
ping God by developing its powers and making it
acquainted with his wonderful and benevolent works,
before we lay down rules of blind obedience.

" Should Laura's life be spared, it is certain she can
be made to understand every religious truth that it may
be desirable to teach her.   Should she die young, there
can be no doubt that she will be taken to the bosom of
that Father in heaven to whom she is every day paying
acceptable tribute of thanksgiving and praise by her
glad enjoyment of the gift of existence.   With these
views, while I am ready to improve every opportunity
of giving what she seems to need, I cannot consent to
attempt to impart a knowledge of any truth for which

her mind is not prepared ; and I would take this opportunity to beseech those friends of hers who differ from me, and who may occasionally converse with her, to reflect that, while the whole responsibility of the case rests upon me, it is unjust in them to do what they may easily do, — instil into her mind notions which might derange the whole plan of her instruction."

CHAPTER VIII.

LAURA has just passed her thirteenth birthday, Dec. 21, 1842, and we turn to the journal to continue our story.

Jan. 2. She was troubled about some little acts of rudeness yesterday, and asked the question, which she so often does now when told she has not done right, " Can God see it and know it, and does he like it? " In her lesson she asked of what cheese is made, and how it differs from butter. " What is name of (here she made a sign of moving her arms up and down) to make butter called? I churned when I lived with my mother, and blistered my hands, and made them very hard. What is chalk? What is ink? What would it do if I drink it, and what would chalk do if I ate it? " Told her it was sometimes taken for medicine. She asked, " Why did not Catherine take chalk? She was sick eight weeks, fifty-six days." She had been told it was New Year's Day yesterday, so to-day she asked, " Is it Happy New Year to-day? Who told all folks it was Happy New Year? "

Jan. 5. Last evening when I returned from Boston I went to the parlor and found Miss J. alone ; soon Laura came in and seated herself, without speaking to any one, at some little distance from either of us.

After sitting quietly knitting for a quarter of an hour she said, " Who talks with you? I think it is Swift." She had been told that I was away, and had no possible way of knowing any one was in the room, except by the motion of the air made in talking, for I had not moved from my chair since she came into the room. Miss J. asked her how she knew any one was in the room. She replied, " I felt them talk."

Jan. 6. Laura had a nervous day, and lost part of her lesson. Talking about some things which she had done in the morning, she said, " What made me very rude? I think I did not feel good in heart, because I broke knob this morning." Asked her if she felt good now. " I cannot feel good until I learn to be good."

It is necessary to explain here our use of the word *rude*, which, perhaps, had acquired a meaning somewhat peculiar. As has been said, Laura has a highly nervous temperament, and while the ceaseless activity which results from it, giving her mind unusual power, is a very valuable assistance in her intellectual training, the effects of it in other directions are to be counteracted constantly. Some days she seems to be in a quiver of nervous excitement, and if we did not resort to systematic exercise and so work off the superfluous nervous fluid, she would have many more such times of trial as that alluded to above. We call all these developments *rudeness*, though, strictly speaking, many of them would not be so considered in the ordinary acceptation of the word.

Laura sometimes showed a little of the coquette which was very amusing. Charles Sumner was, at this time, a frequent visitor, and she felt very well acquainted with him, and was fond of having a play with him occasionally.

Jan. 9. She wished to talk of the gentlemen she had seen lately, and was disposed to criticise them quite severely. " Sumner is not gentle like Doctor. Why does Doctor want Sumner to come here if he is not gentle? " In reply I used the word ‘ like ” instead of " love." She corrected me at once, and said, " Like is not love." " It is not different." Explained the use of "like" in this sense, and she said, " I do not like or love Sumner ; I do not care for him. I did not like Dr. Jarvis when he was here, because I did not know him."

Jan. 10. In the midst of a conversation on bread-making, she suddenly changed the subject by asking, "Why does not God want you in heaven now? Does he know what you teach me? Does he know what I think? Do you? Try." And then she held her forehead towards me, that I might read her thoughts. In speaking of her mother, she said, " She came to see me two times." I gave her the word " twice." She asked how many weeks I stayed in Castine, and when told three, said. " Why did you stay thrice? "

Jan. 13. Commenced her conversation by asking, "Is salt made? " She was much interested in an account of it. Her next query was, " How is gravy made? What is sauce made of? What is lead in my pencil? What is oil made of, and hair-oil, and rum, and camphor, and cologne? What would I do if I drank them? " When told that rum would make her sleepy, and she could not walk straight, she said, " 1 was very sick in head last summer, and very sleepy, and walked crooked."

Jan 19. She had found something about Indians in her book, and asked, " Why do they not have houses like us, and why not clothes like us? I think Indians are very poor. Why did not God give poor Indians clothes like us?" Dr. Jarvis came into the room, and she wished me to ask him if he had ever seen Indians. He told her a story of one which pleased her much. " Why were Indians not white like us? Why do they wear blankets? Are they not sorry not to have clothes?" etc., etc.

Jan. 23. A conversation on " noises," made necessary by her making so many of late. She attempted to justify herself by saying, " Some of my noises are not bad, some are pretty noises. 1 must make noises to call some one." Then to divert attention as well as to get information, " Why does wolf make bad noises?" After half an hour's talk she promised to *try* to remember to be quiet, and during the rest of the day she did remember very well. In the latter part of the day she made a noise in a whisper, and said, " That was with my tongue, 1 made your smooth noise."

Jan. 27. After coming into the school-room she sat still a moment. Some one was playing very softly on the organ in the hall above. She asked, " Why does the house shake? What makes organ shake? Does it make a bad loud noise?"

During the last year many persons of distinction in the world of science and letters had visited

Laura, and among the number George Combe, Esq., of Scotland. Much had been said of the importance of carefully recording everything with regard to this peculiar child, as there might otherwise be many things lost, which would be of the greatest value to science. Dr. Howe had long wished that he could employ a teacher who should devote her whole attention to her, but there were no funds that could be so appropriated. Mr. Combe urged that this ought to be done at once, and a gentleman accompanying him offered to assist in defraying the expense. Others joined him, and the work was assigned to the writer.

At once we arranged an order for study, exercise, and work, as follows : From 6.15 to 7 A. M., arithmetic ; breakfast, domestic duties, putting her room in order, etc., until 9, when we had an hour for conversation. At 10 geography ; at 11 writing ; at 12 reading from books to her, with conversation on the subject. The last fifteen minutes of each hour was a recess. At 1 knitting or sewing ; at 2 she joined the blind girls in calisthenic exercises until her dinner. After dinner a long walk, and then knitting until 6. During her walks not a moment was wasted, as leaning on my right arm, giving herself no care of her footing, which she trusted entirely to my guidance, she conversed steadily, unless the condition of the roads made it impossible for my eye to read her fingers and choose the way at the same time. A walk of five miles under such circumstances was no sinecure as may be readily perceived; indeed, it often proved the most difficult part of the day's work.

Of her general knowledge of language at this time, and her ability to use it, the reader of the previous pages can form an idea. Her lessons in arithmetic had been very irregular, and she had had time between them to forget what she had previously learned. Geography was a new study. We had hitherto read very little to her from books, because the time allowed us was so brief.

She had reached a point now when the desultory manner of teaching, that we had of necessity adopted, ought to be exchanged for one of more system. The much-loved hour in which she had been allowed to bring her own subjects for conversation was continued at nine, and she was pleased when told she was to be taught geography. Writing had always given her much trouble. She was very patient when first learning to form the letters, and wrote well, but soon became careless. In her present stage of advance, she is inclined to think all time spent in attention to the details is wasted, and therefore it becomes irksome to her. She is much more willing to give thought to the matter than to the manner of writing, and perhaps she will have the sympathy of many, who quote the saying, "Bad chirography is evidence of a great mind."

When the new arrangement was announced to her she was delighted, and entered upon it with enthusiasm, approving of it all, save that she would have preferred to spend the hour for her work in the afternoon in play or roaming about, and talking with the blind girls.

Jan. 30. We commenced to-day working by the new schedule. Her first lesson in geography was upon the points of the compass. She had some idea of the four cardinal ones, and she learned in addition those between them. She practised writing some of the letters of the alphabet very slowly, for a quarter of an hour, and was allowed to spend the rest of the time in writing her journal.

She has been in the habit of writing daily a short account of the lessons which have specially interested her, or of any particular incident.

Jan. 31. Wishing to find just what she knew in arithmetic, I gave her an example in addition which she did very well, then in subtraction, when she failed in writing the numbers correctly and in performing the operation. In multiplication she did well. The rest of the lesson was devoted to numeration, writing numbers, and teaching her the hard words of the table. Finding she understood the points of the compass, and could point in any direction I required, after having been placed with her face to the north, I gave her an exercise in bounding the room we were in, and others

round it. I asked her what I meant by " bound." She
took up a piece of india-rubber and throwing it on the
desk said, " It is little elastic and bounds." Had to
explain to her the other signification of the word.

Feb. 1. Found that she could not bound the rooms
I gave her yesterday, unless she went into them. Exercised her in it for some time, and then she bounded the
dining-room and kitchen without going to them ; the
entries were more difficult, but she succeeded in bounding two of them.

I read to her the following story yesterday : —

" 1. An old man had a plum-tree, and when the
plums were ripe he said to his boy. John,

" 2. I want you to pick the plums off my tree, for I
am an old man, and I cannot get up into my tree to
pick them.

" 3. Then John said, ' Yes, sir, I will get up into
the tree and pick them for you.'

" 4. So the boy got up, and the old man gave him a
pail to put the plums in, and he hung it up in the tree
near him.

" 5. And then he put the plums into the pail, one by
one, till the pail was full.

" 6. When the boy saw that the pail was full he said
to the old man, ' Let me give you the pail, for it is full.'

" 7. Then the man held up his hand and took the
pail of plums and put them in his cart.

" 8. ' For,' said he, ' I am to take them to town in
my cart to sell them,' and he gave the boy back the
pail to fill with more plums.

" 9. At last the boy said, ' I am tired and hot ; will
you give me a plum to eat ? '

" 10. ' Yes,' said the old man, ' for you are a good boy, and have worked well; so I will give you ten plums, for you have earned them.'

" 11. The boy was glad to hear him say so, and said, ' I do not want to eat them all now; I will eat five, and take five home to my sister.'

" 12. ' You may get down now,' said the old man, ' for it will soon be dark, and then you will lose your way home.'

" 13. So the boy got down and ran home, and felt glad that he had been kind to the old man.

" 14. And when he got home he was glad he had been kind to his sister, and kept half his plums for her."

To-day she asked me if she might write this story in her journal. The following is a copy of what she wrote without assistance, the punctuation marks alone being added : —

'' An old man had a large plum-tree ; he had a little boy John ; the man asked John to please to go up on the tree to pick many plums, because he was very old and lame. The man gave John a pail for plums. John put them in till it was very full ; he said to the man, it is very full of plums. He took the pail up in his cart to sell them. John was tired & hot ; he asked the man if he might take one plum. The man said he might take ten plums, because he was a very good boy to earn them hard. The man told him to hurry home. He ate five plums ; he gave his sister five plums ; he felt very happy because he helped the old man much, and made his sister happy. John was kind to help the old man ; he was very generous to give his sister part

of his plums. The old man loved John very much.
If John did not hurry home he would have lost the
way. John liked to help the old man well."

The last two or three lines were her own reflections
upon the story.

Feb. 2. She asked me if she was good yesterday.
Told her yes, she had been good all the week. She
said, "Did I do any little thing wrong?" Continued
the conversation on trades, and taught her the word
"furniture"; when I was telling her what work milliners did, she asked, "Do milliners make stockings?
Milliners make stockings that have flowers on them."
In the geography lesson she asked me to teach her
"above," meaning the chambers. She bounded all
the rooms on the second floor, and remembered all of
yesterday's lessons without going to the rooms. In
writing, gave her a lesson in using chalk on the black-
board, but she does not succeed so well as Oliver. At
twelve told her about seeds, and said I would tell her
what her father did (he was a farmer). "How do you
know what my father does? Does your father do so?"
"No; my father is a doctor." "Why is not my father
a doctor? He gave me medicine once, was he a
doctor?"

Feb. 3. Gave her examples in numeration, in hundreds and thousands, which she performed very well,
numerating correctly until she had the number 8,500,
which she wrote 8,050. She hesitated, and then said,
"I think it is wrong"; but it took her a long time to
find how to alter it; when she at length succeeded, she
said, "I was very sad not to know." She asked what
cups and plates and saucers were, and learned the new

word " crockery." " What are rings and knives and
forks?" " Jewelry" and " cutlery" were then learned,
and she brought her work-box for me to tell her of what
it was made. Told her about the pearl with which it is
inlaid, and the rosewood. Then she asked of what
wood the doors were made, and why pineapples were
pine. " Who makes brass hinges for doors?" Talked
about her locket, asked what color it was under the
glass. Being told black, she asked, " How can folks
see through black?" In geography, she bounds any of
the rooms after a moment's thought, and seems to understand it perfectly. She bounded the house, with a little
help. Talked with her about the Point, to try to give
her an idea of it, but failed.

While practising on her letters in writing she does
very well, but as soon as she begins to write in her
journal she is careless again. In the afternoon, she
was asked to go to the school-room to see a committee
of gentlemen, and amused herself while there by asking
the denominations after millions. Setting up a row
of types the whole length of her board, on numerating she found it was eighty quintillions. She asked,
" What people lived eighty quintillions of miles off? I
think it would take ladies a year to go so very far."

Feb. 4. A crowded exhibition. Laura did well,
though at times much excited.

The first Saturday afternoon of each month was
at this time devoted to a public exhibition. For
the first hour Laura was expected to be in the
school-room. As her fame was widespread, there
were usually several hundreds of people present

who wished to see her, and enjoy also the concert by the blind. This was a very trying ordeal, and she often became so much excited (probably in part sympathizing with her teacher) that it was necessary to take a longer walk than usual in preparation for it.

Feb. 6. She writes numbers as high as millions correctly. Took her to the piazza to see the ice and snow; she felt the zinc plates in the lower panes of the windows, and this suggested a lesson on the metals. When talking of iron, she said, "God made some nails, and men made some of iron." She talked about a point, and asked me if I had ever seen a pond. She gave me a description of one and of a river which she said "Tenny taught me about river before I came here, and I threw stones into it." Taught her what an ocean is. When talking of birds, I found she supposed they had four legs, and when I corrected her she asked, "Why did God not give them four?"

Feb. 8. Continued the description of house building from yesterday. She had many questions to ask. "How can men reach to put up the very high posts? How can they fix beams? Where can men sleep when they are building the house? How do carpenters and masons know when to come? How did they learn to build houses? Why do they put fence round the piazzas, and why marble floors?" In geography, when explaining islands to her, she said laughing, "Eyes are very full of tears: are they islands?"

Dr. Howe wished me to try some experiments in teaching her to speak words with her mouth.

Some time ago she happened to make a noise that sounded like ship. I told her she said "ship," and she remembered it always after, and liked to have me ask her to say it. At another time she said "pie," and at another still "doctor." These she constantly used, and has continued to do so all her life. After much labor she said "pa" and "ma" very well, and sometimes succeeded in saying "Abby" and "baby." After trying some time, one day she said, "My mother was wrong to make me deaf." Told her sickness made her so, and she seemed satisfied, but some time after said, "1 am very sad that 1 cannot hear and speak and see," though the next moment she was laughing heartily.

Feb. 9. When checked in making noises she replied, " I only made your noise with my lips, and I tried to talk with my mouth and say Swift, as you and many folks do." In geography she had her first lesson on one of the maps prepared in raised lines for the use of the blind, "Boston and Vicinity." She found South and East Boston and the bridges, and then studied the city itself. She had not known before that streets had names, and was much interested in tracing Washington Street, etc. Had a long talk on the subject of house-building, and how fires sometimes burned them; what people ought to do to save their clothes, etc. She was much excited.

Feb. 10. She told me that she had seen her father " burn short trees" in the ground, meaning stumps 1 presume, and asked why he wanted to do it. From time to time some conversation seems to suggest things which she knew about when living at home, and we see by her questions how much she observed and thought wonderingly about. She seems to have grasped numeration now, so advanced her to addition, which she does perfectly well, but I wished her to understand the reason of carrying to the next column. She learned it very readily. On her map to-day she found all the places she was told yesterday, and learned the names of some of the islands in the harbor, but preferred to move her fingers over the whole map rather than attend to one place.

Feb. 13. Her examples in arithmetic pleased her much, and she found how far from Portland, Me., to Savannah, Ga., by adding the distances between the cities on the route ; how many times the clock strikes in twenty-four hours, etc. In her journal she wrote the following account of a story I read to her yesterday :

" A poor little girl was sitting on the step. A man was passing in the cart and little girl did not know what was in the cart. A man stopped by her and took out a lamb that was almost dead ; he told her she might have it if she wanted it. She held it and kept it warm with her dress, and tried to have it drink some of her milk. It lay down stiff and could not move to drink some milk. It got well after a few days. In one day the little girl lost a lamb and she went to look for it in the barn, but it was not there : then she went to look for it in the wood-yard. She called it to come to her, but it cried because it was very much hurt with a stick of wood. She took the stick from her poor leg. She took

10

it in her arms to get it well. She put it in some soft hay under the sun to go to sleep, and then it could play and frisk."

It was my rule to read a story to her only once, explaining any words that were new, and on the following day she wrote what she could remember in such words as she pleased, and often they were quite unlike the book.

Feb. 14. Laura was left alone with the map, and when I returned said, " I have read all the names and studied Quincy Bay." With very little assistance she bounded Roxbury, Brookline, and Brighton. She now keeps the run of the day of the month, and writes it at the head of each journal entry. Read a story to her which was told as a dialogue ; her account of it was strangely mixed and without sense.

Feb. 16. Gave Laura, among other examples, one requiring her to find the weight of a cow ; when I gave her the weight of the *hide*, I asked her if she knew what I meant. " Yes, to put away things." Taught her " dry measure." Took half a peck of beans and a half-pint measure, told her the number of gills in it, and then had her measure by the cupful, telling me each one how many gills and pints it made, and then at another time the quarts, pints, and gills, until she had measured the half-peck. Such lessons are her delight, and she was very soon entirely familiar with it, and could quickly answer questions on the number of gills or pints in a peck, bushel, etc. I copy the story alluded to above, as she wrote it after the second reading :

"One day little Rollo was sitting by the fire on his green cricket; his mother was sitting at her work-table; he asked her, 'When father would come home?' She said, 'He will come pretty soon.' Rollo told her he thought he had better go and take hold of the great rocking-chair to pull it to the fire for father. So he began to cry because chair would not come to the fire to please him. Mother looked up, — 'Rollo, what is the matter?' and he said, 'The chair will not come.' Mother said, 'Why Rollo wanted it?' He said he 'Wanted to save father the trouble.'" (This was a phrase she had lately learned, so she used it here, although not in the story.) "She told Rollo that he troubled her by crying; then he stood by the chair and swang back and forth. By and by, he said he was going to get his father's slippers from the little closet by the side of the fire and put them in the corner by the fire. When his father came home, then Rollo ran to the door, and said to him he could not move the chair, but father's slippers are all ready for him."

Feb. 17. One example in arithmetic this morn was, to find the age of a man, having the time he had lived in several places given. She said, "He lived in many places, I am not sure why, — why?" She asked many questions about a party I attended last evening, "How the ladies knew when to come?" Taught her "invitation." "Why was not I invited?" Told her she was a little girl. "Doctor says I am tall." But she was satisfied when told that the blind girls did not go. She was much amused in her walk yesterday over snow that was incrusted, but not sufficiently to bear her weight. When she broke through, she would scream

with delight, and pull me after her. Promised to
explain the reason in the lesson this morning, so we
talked on ice, etc.

Found to my surprise that she could bound all the
towns I had taught her without the aid of the map, and
to-day she completed the circuit of Boston from Roxbury round to Malden. She takes much pleasure in
this study.

At noon took her to the stable to let her measure
oats with the half-peck measure, and then to the store-
room to teach her wine measure. Found a gallon, and
also hogshead, tierce, and barrel. She readily learned
their names and number of gallons they would hold, and
then wanted to examine other things, — coffee in a bag,
sugar and salt in barrels, ginger, pepper, etc., in boxes
of twenty-five pounds, starch in papers, tea-chest box
and lead within. It was my intention to make two lessons of this, but there was no place to stop answering
her questions.

Feb. 18. When she bounded Chelsea, and found it
was north by Reading, she said, "Who lives in Reading?" making the sign of reading in a book, and laughing heartily.

The following is a copy of a letter written in place of
her journal exercise : —

TWENTYTH DAY OF FEBRUARY.

MY DEAR MISS SUSAN :

Miss Swift sends much love to you, & she wants
to see you. Miss Swift teaches me five hours, — to
cypher, & to talk about many things, and to study
geography, & to write & to read about stories in the
books to me. She teaches me calisthenics every day in

the afternoon. Will you please to write a letter to me some time? I was very sore from exercising; I am well now. I send my love to Mrs. Swift; I want to see her very much. I like calisthenics much; it makes me strong and well, like the walking. I go to meeting with Miss Rogers every Sunday. I like to go to meeting very much. Good by, my friend.

Feb. 22. Found that she was studying her geography with a thorough understanding of it. Some days since she had learned to bound West Cambridge; and to-day, when asked to bound Lexington, she traced it on the map until she got to the south, and then took off her hands and said, "I must *think* the south," and in an instant told me, "By West Cambridge."

Dr. Howe thus relates the story of deception which occurred this day, prefacing it with the remark that it was perhaps attributable to indiscretion on his part: —

"She came to me one day dressed for a walk, and had on a new pair of gloves which were stout and rather coarse. I began to banter and tease her (in that spirit of fun of which she is very fond, and which she usually returns with interest) upon the clumsy appearance of the hands, at which she first laughed, but soon began to look so serious and even grieved that I tried to direct her attention to something else, and soon forgot the subject. But not so poor Laura; here her personal vanity or her love of approbation had been wounded; she thought the gloves were the cause of it, and she resolved to be rid of them. Accordingly, they disap-

peared and were supposed to be lost; but her guileless
nature betrayed itself, for without being questioned she
frequently talked about the gloves, not saying directly
that they were lost, but asking if they might not be in
such or such a place. She was uneasy under the new
garb of deceit, and soon excited suspicion. When it
reached my ears, I was exceedingly pained, and, moreover, doubtful what course to pursue. At last, taking
her in the most affectionate way, I began to tell her a story
of a little girl who was much beloved by her parents
and brothers and sisters, and for whose happiness everything was done; and asked her whether the little girl
should not love them in return and try to make them
happy, to which she eagerly assented. But, said I,
she did not; she was careless and caused them much
pain. At this, Laura was excited, and said the girl
was in the wrong, and asked what she did to displease
her relations. I replied, she deceived them. They
never told her anything but truth; but she, one day,
acted so as to make them think she had not done a
thing, when she had done it. Laura then eagerly asked
if the girl told a fib, and I explained to her how one
might tell a falsehood without saying a word, which she
readily understood, becoming all the time more interested and evidently touched. I then tried to explain
to her the different degrees of culpability. resulting
from carelessness, from disobedience, and from inten-
tional deceit. She soon grew pale, and evidently
began to apply the remarks to her own case, but still
was very eager to know about "*the wrong little girl*,"
and how her parents treated her. I told her her parents
were grieved and cried, at which she could hardly

restrain her own tears. After a while, she confessed
to me that she had deceived about the gloves, that they
were not lost, but hidden away. I then tried to show
her that I cared nothing about the gloves, that the loss
of a hundred pairs would be nothing if unaccompanied
by any deceit. She perceived that I was grieved, and
going to leave her to her own thoughts, clung to me as
if in terror of being alone. I was forced, however, to
inflict the pain upon her.

" Her teachers and the persons most immediately
about her were requested to manifest no other feeling
than that of sorrow on her account; and the poor crea-
ture, going about from one to another for comfort and
for joy, but finding only sadness, soon became agonized
with grief. When left alone, she sat pale and motion-
less, 'with a countenance the very image of sorrow; and
so severe seemed the discipline that I feared lest the
memory of it should be terrible enough to tempt her to
have recourse to the common artifice of concealing one
prevarication by another, and thus insensibly get her
into the habit of falsehood. I therefore comforted her
by assurances of the continued affection of her friends,
tried to make her understand that their grief and her
suffering were the simple and necessary consequences
of her careless or wilful misstatement, and made her
reflect upon the nature of the emotion she experienced
after having uttered the untruth; how unpleasant it
was, how it made her feel afraid, and how widely different it was from the fearless and placid emotion which
followed truth."

Feb. 23. The morning lesson was very good, but at
the hour for conversation she could only talk about the

gloves, and at request of Dr. H. I left her to sit by herself.

Feb. 24. She finished the map of Boston and vicinity. When asked to name the towns north, west, and south of Boston, she did it correctly at once, without reference to the map. She has taken less time on this map than any of the blind children.

Later in the day she asked, " Are you tired to live?" Corrected the form of question, and answered, " No." " Are you tired of moving?" Asked her if she was tired of living. " No, but you have lived many years." " Do you think you would be tired if you had lived twenty years?" She hesitated, and thought some time about it, but decided she should not.

Feb. 25. " When I am a lady I shall go and never come ; Doctor says ladies do not go to school." Asked where she should go. " To Hanover, but I want you to come and live with me to take care of baby sister, because my mother and the girl are very busy, and cannot take care of her and me." " When you are a lady, you ought to take care of yourself." She said, " Can I tell myself when to put on other dress?" She talked a long time about what things she could do to help her mother, and then changed the subject to talk about " giving away things." She said, " Doctor says I must not give things away that ladies give me." Fearing that she had not quite understood his meaning, and that she might think this would be an excuse for selfishness, I proposed that she should give to her little sister the playthings which she did not use now ; she made several excuses for not doing so, but at last concluded she would like to. She said, " Pigs are very stingy, they eat all the food, and do not give baby pigs any." Told her the birds gave each other food. This was a puzzle to her, and she talked long, trying to settle the question if the pigs were wrong. Children usually prefer to skip the moral of a story, but Laura always wishes to discuss it; she never seems quite satisfied with the results of her own reasoning, or with my verdicts on such questions.

Feb. 27. Laura told me a story of her early childhood to-day: "When I was a little girl in Hanover I threw the cat into the fire, and she ran fast, and my mother ran fast to take her out, and she burned her foot very much. She went away into the woods, and never came out." It is singular that, after being with us and able to talk for so many years, she should just now remember an incident of this kind and relate it.

After recess she said, "I was very much frightened. I thought I felt some one make a great noise, and I trembled, and my heart ached very quick." Probably the children had made some unusual sound in romping, but I had not perceived it. She asked, "Do you know any crazzy persons?" Then altered the word to "craxy," and finally "crazy." Asked who told her that word. She said, "Lurena told about crazy persons, and said she was once crazy herself. What is crazy?" Told her crazy persons could not think what they were doing, and attempted to change the subject, but she immediately returned to it, and repeated the question, "Have you seen crazy people?" And would not be satisfied without an answer. I replied, "I saw a woman once who walked about." "Why did she walk? How could she think to walk?" Here she showed the

error of my definition. Explained to her that sometimes people were sick, and that made them crazy.
" Who will take care of me if I am crazy? " Laughed
at her, and told her she would not be. " I said *if.*"
I promised to take care of her if she would be gentle
and kind to me. " Can I talk with my fingers? Did
you ever see a dizzy lady? How do you dizzy? " She
said she dreamed last night about her mother and the
baby, and talked with her fingers as in the daytime.
I questioned her particularly as to what she dreamed,
but got no satisfactory answer.

Laura writes a great many letters to her friends now.
The following is a copy of one just written to her
mother. She has in this for the first time asked questions about family affairs. I asked why she said, " My
dear *my* mother." " She is my mother, and she would
not know if I did not write it so."

My Dear my Mother:

I want to see you very much. I send very much
ove to you. I send ten kisses to sister Mary. My one
pair of stockings are done.* Can Mary walk with her
feet? Do stockings fit her? I want you to write a
letter to me some time. Miss Swift teaches me to say
father, & mother, & baby. I want you to come to
South Boston with my sister, to stay few days and to
see me exercising the calisthenics. Oliver can talk
with his fingers very faster about words. I will write a
letter to you again. Miss J. & Doctor send love to
you. Miss Davis is married, — Mrs. Davis; she has
gone to live with her husband in Dudley. Is Mary well?

---

* She had knit a pair to send with the letter.

Is my aunt well? I send love to her. I will write a letter to you soon some time. Why did you not write a letter to me? I go to meeting every Sunday. I am gentle in church with Miss Rogers. I am happy there. Good-bye.

Feb. 28. Laura was quite forgetful in her lesson, and said as an excuse, " I was thinking about wife and Doctor." She had just been told of Doctor's intended marriage, and evidently did not know whether to be glad or sorry about it. She said, " To-morrow will be March; will it be the once day of March?"

March 1. Taught her cloth measure, and let her measure everything about her. She was quite disturbed to find her fingers were all of different length, and said, " Why did not God make them all alike?" In geography found she had forgotten some of her definitions, so gave her a review, and at its close she answered in her own words all such questions as, What is an island? Cape? Bay? etc. She asked if I would give her the map to-morrow, where the birds canary live. Told her that was very far off, that other little girls did not know that map, but that if she remembered well what I taught her, she would learn it soon.

March 3. She explains the process of multiplication by one figure very well, and seems to understand it perfectly. Found difficulty in deciding on the best map for her to study, as there is none of the State of Massachusetts prepared for the blind, on a sufficiently large scale, and the step from that she has been studying to one on which a pin-head denotes a town, and but few

towns even marked in this way, is a very long one.
Decided upon an outline map. Commenced by telling
her where Boston and Charles River were, and then
attempted to give her the idea that the map was so
small and it had so many miles on it, we could not have
room to put down all that was on the other map. Told
her the number of miles from Boston to the mouth of
the Hudson River. She said, "I think Miss W. lives
there," and was much pleased that she should have
learned anything so far from home.

March 4. The monthly exhibition day. Laura was
puzzled to know why there are sometimes three Satur-
days, and sometimes four between them. It took some
time to explain this.

March 6. Gave her for a writing lesson the story I
had read to her three days before. She thought she
should not be able to remember it, but she did well.
After writing she said, "Is this truth? I think not.
Is it lie?" Tried to make her understand it was not
wrong to write it, but doubt if I succeeded entirely.
In writing she spelled the word "bureau" incorrectly,
and when told of it, said, "I was very unremembered."
She uses "forgetful" often, but this was an effort to
coin a word, and she turned to me for approbation of it.

March 8. The geography lesson was the towns on
the Eastern Railroad, and also on the Lowell and
Providence roads. She enjoyed tracing the routes
which the blind scholars take to go to their homes.

The next lesson was the towns on the coast in Plym-
outh and Barnstable Counties to the extremity of Cape
Cod. When told this name she asked, "To eat?"
The bays and islands, Martha's Vineyard and Nantucket

Interested her, and she was much amused at such names as " Ply-mouth, Barn-stable," etc. She always seems to think of words in their component parts.

March 10. Not quite as good a lesson as usual in arithmetic. She found an algebra type, and was anxious to be able to use it. Told her I would teach her all about it when she was sixteen. " And can you kiss me then? Can you kiss sixteen young ladies?" She expressed much fear that she should have to give up kissing and being kissed when she was so old.

When Laura was having a lesson on a subject in which she was specially interested, she appeared to be in a state of great excitement; each new thought was received with a hearty laugh, or a kiss or a hug for her teacher. The desire to express her delight was irresistible. The question was often asked by visitors, " What is it pleases her so much?" when perhaps it was only a new word which she had learned from a sentence dictated by a stranger, which I had interpreted to her and afterwards explained.

March 11. On some points of etiquette she needs special instruction, and to-day the subject of visiting came up. Sometimes, of late, when asked to call on a person, she has added, " And to take tea?" When told of the impropriety of this, she carried it to the opposite extreme, and thought Miss J. must be to blame when she went to her sister's without an invitation, and questioned whether it was proper for me to pay any calls unless a special invitation to do so was extended; but she at last understood the propriety of thanking people for the invitation, and that she was not to ask for anything more.

She had a story read to her to-day in which was the sentence, " One day John was a little cross." As a comment she said, " I think the man " (who wrote the story) " guessed that." One of the questions in arithmetic was, " If a man travel seven miles an hour, how far will he travel in eight days, when the days are nine hours long? " She did not know the word " travel," so an explanation of that and the word " journey " occupied some time. She performed it correctly, but when asked to explain it, did not succeed. Thought she might do better if I put myself in the place of the man. After thinking a moment she said, " You will have to go more; you will have to go over the bridges." When she found the answer was several hundred miles, she said, " When will you come back? "

Her imagination seemed to develop more slowly than any other power of her mind, and this caused her to meet with difficulties where I have never known any child who could hear to encounter them.

March 13. Laura said on coming down early this morning, " I hope I shall not be cross, or make noises, or fret, or deceive, or tell any wrong stories this week." Taught her the words " resolution " and " resolved," and she understood them both very quickly. She asked a question, which I answered playfully, " Yes, ma'am." Explained the use of " ma'am," and also of " sir." She asked what the punctuation marks meant in her Child's Book. Gave her the names, and attempted to explain them, but it will take much practice before she succeeds in using them correctly. She learned the words " surprise " and " strange." Asked her for illustrations, and she gave the sentence, " I am surprised to know I shall go to the State House."

The exhibition of the pupils of the Institution before the Legislature was always an exciting episode, and although we used the greatest care to keep Laura calm, she sympathized with the family.

March 15. Her mind being entirely occupied with the experience of yesterday, I took the State House and its uses as a subject of conversation. She learned the word " representative " with much difficulty.

March 16. The requests for Laura's autograph were always numerous, and it was often very irksome to her to write. When I asked her to prepare some this morning which Doctor H. wished to use, she objected, and at last with reluctance took her pencil and wrote hurriedly with one hand. I took her hand in mine and told her it made me feel sad to have her do so, and she soon said, " I feel bad in my heart, and that makes me wrong." After a moment's thought she wrote very well.

CHAPTER IX.

March 17. Having devoted six weeks to lessons on written arithmetic, and taught her all the tables of weights and measures which would be of use to her, I decided that she would be better prepared to advance further by studying Colburn's Mental Arithmetic first. I supposed she would be much amused at the simple questions in the first section; when asked how many hands she had, she said, "Two, but I saw Mr. Rogers, who has only one" Her comments on nearly every question were such as, "That boy was very kind and generous. Why did this boy buy much cake?" etc., etc. She, as usual, took every statement as a fact, and the amusement was all on my side. She was much pleased at her success in the gymnasium yesterday, when she swung herself up seven rounds of the ladder. Here she stopped, and I lifted her down. She thought she might go to the top to-day, and wanted to know if she could jump to the floor. Showed her the pole near by for her to cling to and slide down, but she was afraid to attempt it. I can talk to the blind girls and encourage them while they are attempting new feats, but poor Laura has both hands in use, and it is not a cause of wonder that she is timid, but rather that she accomplishes so much.

March 18. She enjoys her mental arithmetic, as she

can answer the questions so easily. She said, "I think I am very bright this morning, I have done many sums." On the map she has learned all the principal towns in the east of New England, and to-day learned those between Worcester and the Connecticut River. Her memory is wonderful, as she rarely forgets one of the names given her.

March 20. She performed thirty examples, and gave the reasons for her work. This she dislikes, and says, " I never did tell why before, and why do you have me now?" At nine she brought "The Child's Second Book" and asked that she might read to me. I found her yesterday puzzling over it, and when I spoke to her, she said, " I cannot read books and know them as you do." Again she had found that unfortunate sentence which had so grieved her a year ago, and to-day it is a discouragement to me, for I supposed she would now read it, as she should, connectedly, but find I am mistaken. " You must not think because you are blind, you cannot learn as much as other children." Again she stops at the comma and says, " Cannot I think? Why did Dr. Howe say I could not?"

March 22. She was puzzled by a question in arithmetic this morning, " What will a gallon of molasses cost at two cents a gill?" but succeeded at last in doing it without assistance. She enjoyed a review in geography, as I made a play of going from town to town in Massachusetts, and having her tell what places we would pass through, having her tell me also the direction in which she was travelling. It seems to me that few children make a geography lesson so completely their own as she does. She did not appear well after her walk, and

11

said, " I must ask doctor why my blood is cold, and does not run about and be warm as J.'s." She found in her book the word "syllable." I do not like to tell her she cannot understand a word, it makes her so sad, so told her what I could of this way of dividing words, but it is so dependent upon the ear that I do not think she can ever be taught it, so she can use it.

March 27. A lesson on halves which took an hour : but I hope the way is prepared for thirds, etc. When I called her to come for a lesson, she said, " I have been reading about God." Asked if she understood all the words ; she said, " No, I thought I would wait patient until you were not busy."

March 30. Read the following to her, " If you can buy a barrel of cider for four dollars, how much can you buy for one dollar?" Her comments were, " How did the man who wrote the book know I was here?" and " I cannot give much for cider, because it is very sour." Fractions prove very puzzling to her. Our walk to-day was from the Institution to the lower part of Mt. Vernon Street, round the Common and home, which took nearly three hours, but she did not seem tired. She asked how candy was made. Found she did not know what raisins are made from, so we had a lesson on vineyards, etc., and she learned the new word " shrivelled."

March 31. When in a shop in Boston she showed some impatience on being checked in making a noise, and perceiving that I had in my hand a bundle of muslin which I wished to keep smooth, she pinched it very hard. On leaving the shop I told her I could not talk with her because she had done wrong, and asked if she knew in what. "Yes, I pinched your cloth." And we walked on silently. As we were crossing the bridge, there was a sail-boat so near, that by extending her arm I could put her hand upon the sail. I stopped to let her examine it, but she did not talk about it. When we got home, she said, "Do you feel sad? Why did you let naughty girl feel of the boat?" Told her I did not like to punish her, and I thought she would want to feel it very much. This touched her feelings, and she was very sad and thoughtful all the forenoon.

These little bursts of anger were very slight, and perhaps many would say it is not just to mention them at all. Were I writing of any ordinary child, I should not do so, but in giving these notes to the world, it seems to be my duty to tell of things just as they happened whether they were large or small.

April 3. Last evening when walking with Laura, we met Oliver. She said to him, "Laura is sick." I asked where, as I had not noticed it. "In my head, I studied much in books, and thought very hard." (Sunday afternoon when she was left alone.) Found she had been studying in "Viri Romæ," and she remembered several words, "non, sed, est," etc., and was anxious to know what they meant. When told, she asked, "Does Doctor know Latin, and Jeannette and Rogers and Sophia?" And when she found some did not, she was very happy. "Does God know Latin? Do you know all things like God?" The occasional glimpses which she gets of the world of letters beyond discour-

age her at first, and she seeks companions in her ignorance, but they serve in the end only to whet her curiosity. She had also found many other new English
words to ask about. "What is England? Is Doctor
going there? What does 'altered her mind' mean?
Are snatch and scratch the same? What is education?"
She had an idea, from some reason unknown to me,
that this was a French word. "Do French people say
they will education children?" Taught her the verb
"educate."

April 10. Gave her a lesson on a large map of the
New England States, and she found the towns upon it
with ease. At noon told her she might think of a subject for our lesson, and when I returned she said, "Talk
about Jupiter." She was satisfied when told it was the
name of a star, and asked, "What does orbit mean?"
Then she talked of the wind; when told that it blew
northeast and was very cold, and yesterday it was south
and very warm, she asked, "Is the wind always south
in summer? Will you teach me next summer and winter, and after two summers?" "Perhaps the Doctor
will think you had better go home, and help your mother
make cheese and butter." She showed much adroitness
in settling the moral questions which I knew would be
raised at once by the suggestion, and answered, "Doctor says he wants me to live with him, and I think my
sister will help my mother."

April 12. She wished to write a note of thanks to a
gentleman who had sent her some candy, and came to
me in trouble because she did not know how to address
it. "I cannot say My *dear* Mr. Howard." When
told she could say simply, "Mr. Howard," she was

much relieved. No one had ever made a suggestion of this kind to her, but her delicate sense of propriety never fails her. She had tried to speak my name with her mouth. I found the combination of consonants too difficult, and suggested that she try to speak " Mary." She succeeded very well, but to-day said, " I am little afraid to say ' Mary.' I think other folks would think it was their name." She asked if she had been very gentle this week. "Yes, I think so." But she was not satisfied. " I think I was a little cross yesterday in arithmetic: my forehead was wrinkled." She went with me to a shop to select a collar. Before going in I told her they did not like to have them touched much, but that she could feel of the one I bought. She kept her hands very still for some time, and then I showed her one I liked. She said, " I think I could find you a very pretty one," and in a moment selected a very fine one. The salesman, wishing to know if she would manifest any more pleasure at the finest work, showed her one of the most costly he had. She felt of it carefully, and said, " That is very, very beautiful, and I think it is velvet." She had many questions to ask about embroidery of all kinds to-day.

April 17. A question in her arithmetic lesson to-day was, " There is a vessel containing eighty-seven gallons, and by a cock, ten gallons run into it in an hour. in how many hours will it be filled?" She said, " How can gallons run?" She associated the word " run " with the measure I had shown her when she first learned it, but when I added, " of wine or water," she understood it. At noon, I told her she might sweep ıe stairs to help Ellen. This was quite a trial for her, as she is not very fond of domestic work, and she wanted a story read to her at this hour, but she came out of it nobly. At first she looked displeased, then her countenance brightened, and she said, " Yes, I can sweep for money, because I am very poor without money." Told her she must sweep them to try to pay Ellen and J. for doing work for her, and that she did not do anything for them, but they worked much for her. After a moment's thought, she kissed me, and said, " Yes, I will go and try to do them well, that I may pay J. and Ellen for many nice things." And she did them faithfully, though it occupied her two hours.

April 18.   Completed the third section of Colburn's Mental Arithmetic. Her lesson in geography was on New Hampshire. She is familiar with its large towns, rivers, lakes, and mountains. Showed her where her mother lived, and talked about the college, why called Dartmouth, etc. Continued reading a story which was commenced a fortnight since, but she could tell me just where we left it.

April 20.   Laura said to me last eve, " I do not *think* now, I dream." I supposed she was joking, and took little notice of it, but this morning she asked, " Why could I not think last night?" " I think you did." " No, I only dreamed, I did not know anything well." She expressed much sorrow about Doctor's going away, and perhaps this was the cause of her peculiar state.

April 21.   A beautiful spring day, so took Laura out to the play-ground for a lesson on trees; taught her about the evergreens, and showed her the buds just swelling on the other trees. Then she visited the pigpen, tried to get the cat to come to her, and when she succeeded, I held her so she could feel her head, ears, nose, and mouth. She has always before shrunk from touching her, but she has known of Julia Brace's * affection for cats, and I think this made her less timid. She felt of its whiskers, and at once said that was what Julia meant by her sign for a cat. When told its eyes were green, she said, " I think they are very beautiful." She was so happy that she laid her plans for taking all her lessons next summer in the arbor. In geography she surprised me more than ever, by learning the names and situation of Lake Champlain and four rivers running into it, and of about ten towns in Vermont, afte*** I had spelled them only once to her.

April 24. She asked for a lesson in the china closet, that she might learn the names of different pieces of china and glass. In the fourth section of the arithmetic she has done, in two mornings, over fifty such sums as. " Three times seven are how many times four? "

April 25. Found her too much engaged with her cares as housekeeper, which she has assumed in Miss J.'s absence, to attend to a lesson. She had cleared two closets of their contents and wished to be allowed to complete her cleaning. She could tell me in her geography lesson the names of the cities through which Miss J. passed in going to New York.

April 26. Laura said this morning, " My heart ached, I was very much frightened last night. 1 do not know what made my blood make a noise." Told her I

---

* This deaf. dumb, and blind woman. whose home was in Hartford Ayslum for Deaf-Mutes, had been at South Boston for some weeks.

thought she dreamed. "I did not know that dream could make my heart afraid. I put sheet over my head very quick; I trembled very much." "I dream sometimes and am frightened." "When your dream frightens you. do you think you feel some one walking?" At breakfast she asked each person she met, if her dreams ever frightened her. "What shall I do if I am frightened?" "Laugh, to think that you dreamed." At nine she could think of nothing else. "When I was at Halifax with you and Miss J., I came from my bed because I was frightened." Told her I sometimes dreamed of falling. "I do sometimes, and then I make a noise and jump. I think dream was very hard and heavy and thick; it made me grow quick, my blood ran very hard." "I think you dreamed that some one was walking and that frightened you." "Did some one walk?" "No." "Did you think you *heard* some one" (here she corrected me and said felt) "walk after you woke, or did you remember feeling them before you woke?" "I felt them and woke very quick, my eyes opened very quickly. What made my blood run very noise?" (Here she made a low noise.) "I thought something had four legs, and it ran almost over me." She was so much excited about it that I tried to laugh it off, but she seemed to think it was nothing to joke about. "I can come to you when I am frightened?" "Yes, and I can wake you and tell you it is all a dream, and you can laugh and go to sleep again." Then it seemed as if she had just remembered what her dream was, for I had asked her several times before, and said, "I dreamed last night that Wight came to my room with a pig, and that the pig ran down hill on a

board to my bed." " Was this what frightened you? "
" Yes."

April 28. She performed thirty examples in an
hour, such as the following : " Eight times seven and
two sevenths of seven are how many times nine? " She
had her first lesson on Maine ; when told the name of
the capital, she said, laughing, " Is it a little girl? "
She talked much of Doctor's wedding, and said, " I
wanted to go to see Doctor wedding. Do ladies wear
very nice dresses? Did Doctor wear very nice? When
you are married I shall come to your wedding, and
wear very nice silk," then changed her sentence, saying, " I meant *if.*" She sat still an unusually long
time, and I asked what she was thinking about. " I
love Doctor, like Mrs. Howe. I love him very, very
much ; is he my daughter? He said he was." " I think
he said you were his daughter, did he not? " " Is Mrs.
Howe my sister? " " If Doctor is your father, then she
will be your mother." " No ; J. is mother. I cannot
love Mrs. Howe as I do J., because I do not see her
often ; she is a stranger."

April 29. She went yesterday to visit the steamship
in which the Doctor was to sail for Europe. She examined the saloon, the tables, felt of the glasses in the
racks, and then visited the state-rooms and cabins.
After seeing the crockery she said, " I have seen cups
and saucers and plates ; where are spoons and knives
and forks? Will you show me where men keep the
'our and molasses? " Bread and molasses is her favorite dish. Next she asked to see where they cooked,
and wanted to know if men could make things good.
The cook happened to be near, and, to prove his abil-

ity, gave her a cake; and then she asked where cakes stay (were kept). "Where do men get milk to make cakes?" She was taken to see the cow. Lastly she walked the whole length of the ship, to get an idea of its size.

May 9. She was very much excited, so tried to interest her in a talk about the weather, and why she could feel the storm from some of the windows, and not from the others, but she was unable to fix her attention. She was inclined to conceal her own sadness at parting with Dr. Howe, who sailed to-day, and said to me when she had been to say good by, "Do not be very sad, I will make you happy." I brought Oliver into our rooms, thinking that talking with him might amuse her, and make him feel more happy. She said, "I will try very hard to make him happy. He must not be sad." She led him to Doctor's chamber to show him that all the things were taken away, and talked with him till dinner. After this she became more quiet.

May 2. She completed an unusually long letter to her friend, Miss Everett. She said, "I must write a very long letter to her, because she has not been here for very long time, and she will want to know about all things, and it will make her happy." It is much the most gossiping letter she ever wrote, so I copy it entire:—

FIRST OF MAY.

MY DEAR ELIZABETH EVERETT:

I want to see you very much. I have not seen you for very many months. You did not write a letter to me for very long time. Why did you not write to me? I send very much love to you. I am sad that you did never come to see us last summer, to stay a few days. Are you very well? I am well. Were you sad not to come to S. Boston? Mrs. Morton has got baby named Lucy. I & Miss J are going to see Mrs. M. & little baby next summer & to pick berries. Dr. went to New York to see Miss Ward many times because he loved her very much. Last Saturday morning he went to New York to be married Wednesday evening. Miss Ward is married, — Mrs. Howe. Miss J. went to see Dr. married Wednesday evening. Mrs. H. came with her husband to stay till Monday. Before dinner they are going in ship to stay two weeks. I went to see ship Friday, where (in which) Dr. is going away. I went with Miss S. & Miss R. & Miss W. & Oliver & Mr. H. & Mrs. S. to see ship, & cups, and saucers, and plates, & many glass tumblers, & berths, & other things. I am very sad to have Dr. & Mrs. Howe go & stay many months, one year. They will go three thousand miles, far off. My very dear lame friend sends much love to you. Mrs. Howe can talk with her fingers, she goes away in May. Will you please to write a letter to me some time? Miss S. sends her love to you. Dr. & Mrs. Howe went away in the ship Monday. They will come next spring, very long. I went to (visit) Mrs. B. before dinner till night. I had a very pleasant time. I was happy there last Thursday. Miss S. teaches me five hours, — to cypher, & to talk, & to study geography well, & to write, & to read to me in books about very pretty stories. It is vacation now. I want to come to see you. Miss Davis is married, Mrs. Davis has gone to live with her husband. All the girls are very well & good.   Goodbye.

It is quite touching to see how the thought of
Dr. Howe as just going, and then as gone, and
then not to return for so long a time, runs like a
sad refrain all through the letter.   Few children
would have borne such trials as bravely as she
did.

May 4.   She asked why I hurried in sewing, and
when told because I had much to do and very little
time to do it in, said, " I can hem handkerchiefs for
you," and this afternoon has worked very diligently all
the time, though she had work of her own which she
wished to do.

May 5.   She completed the fourth section in arithmetic, and after that could talk of nothing but the
vacation.   As I was to be absent three weeks from her,
she wished to be told what she could do every day, and
almost every hour.   She seems to prefer to lean on me,
rather than to be independent as so many girls of her
age wish to be.

May 31.   Laura was very happy to welcome the
blind girls on their return.   She busied herself in assisting me in arranging my room, and as she knows the
place for everything in my bureau drawers, she can be
very useful.   She was anxious to tell me of all that had
happened in the vacation, and to hear what I had been
doing.   Being "anniversary week," we had a large
number of visitors, so had only time to ask questions
on the map of New England.   She had just completed
it and was very ready in answering questions a month
ago, and I was anxious to test her memory.   Found
she remembered much of it, and probably a few days of

review will bring it all back. On returning from our walk we met in the hall a little blind girl who was a new scholar. Thinking it would please her, I stopped for her to feel of her, but she treated her rather roughly. This afternoon the little girl sent her an orange. I said that I thought she was very kind and had forgiven her rudeness in the morning. She made no reply, but I could see that she appreciated the reproof intended.

June 1. She brought some candy and said, " I want you to give them to little Jane, and tell her I thank her for the orange very much." Found, in a review of four States, she had forgotten only three places. Some one had been talking to her about monkeys, and she wished to repeat to me the stories. The way in which they were made to throw down cocoa-nuts from the trees amused her, but the question whether it was right (morally) for the men to throw stones at the monkeys was raised at once.

She has forgotten more in her arithmetic than in anything else, which I regret, as she is always more easily troubled by failures and enjoys the study less than any other. When discouraged she often says, " It is very hard, I think I cannot know it."

It generally happened that her times of greatest trouble came very unexpectedly, and when her previous conversation would have led me to anticipate an unusual amount of self-restraint. An example of this occurred

June 7. She asked, " Was I good all day yesterday?" " Nearly all day ; you were rude two or three times." ' It makes me sad in eyes, and something troubles me when I am not good." She had commenced a new section in arithmetic and was puzzled but in very good spirits. She tried unsuccessfully to tell me how much a quarter of eight was, and said, "I do not know." I replied, as I always do when she does not take time, " If you think, you can tell me." Instead of receiving it as usual, she caught my hand and twisted it very hard. At first I thought it was play and was surprised to see her face was scarlet, and that she was in a passion. I left my seat beside her without speaking, and she sat alone a quarter of an hour. Then I went to her to tell her it was time for her to put her room in order. When I went to take her to breakfast she said, " I think you do not want very angry girls to eat with you ; you can bring my breakfast, and I can eat alone." Told her I liked to have her go with me. When she came for her next lesson, I asked her if she felt happy. " No, I was very angry. I twisted your hand and almost broke your wrist. Does it ache now ? " Told her I was very sad that she felt so, and asked her if I was unkind to her. " You told me to think." Explained why I said so, and that I could not teach her well unless she took time to think. She said, " You were kind, but I was angry. What will you do to punish me ? " " Nothing, I do not want to punish you." " You did punish me very much when I sat alone." " If you had been good you would not care if I left you alone ; it is your thoughts that punish you and make you sad and unhappy." " What will you do to punish me if I am angry again ? " " Nothing. I shall be kind to you, and try to teach you, but I am afraid if you are angry I cannot love you so much as I do when you are mild and gentle, and it makes me very sad to have you so." She wiped her tears, and thinking of some work she could do to help Miss J., I sent her to do it, hoping to change the current of her thoughts. All the rest of the day she was very affectionate, and frequently said, " You are very kind to me," as if trying to make me forget the morning.

June 8. She asked if " think, guess, suppose, and understand " are the same. An hour was too short to make her fully understand the difference ; indeed, I doubt whether any explanations, illustrations, etc., will avail, but she must learn their exact meaning as other children do, by having them used constantly in conversation with her.

Her geography lesson was on the large map of the United States. She was already so ·familiar with New England that she soon adjusted herself to the new scale of distances, etc., and one lesson sufficed. Passing her hand over all the great map, she said, " I cannot learn so very much, I cannot remember." A few weeks since she had a lesson in the play-ground, and to-day she felt of what were then little buds, and was delighted to find not only leaves but flowers on the trees and plants. She learned many new names.

June 9. This morning she did not feel very friendly towards Mr. Warren Colburn ; she asked, " Why does man put sums in book for girls to guess? " After studying some time on one she said, " I am not very widsom. What does widsom mean? To know much like Doctor? " Taught her the noun " wisdom " and the adjective " wise," and encouraged her by telling her that Doctor had to study such sums when he was a little boy, to make him very wise. While talking about Eastern New York with the map before her, she stopped to ask, " Do you want to see God? Do you want Him

to want you now? Does He see us, does He know what
I say to you? Do you think of Him? Do all people
love God? How many bodies has God made? Ten
thousand billion?" Her lesson led to the subject of
canals, and we had a long talk about the Erie Canal
and Niagara Falls. It might be supposed that they
would be mere commonplace topics to her, and that the
most vivid description could not convey to one, who had
never even seen water, the faintest idea of their beauty
and grandeur. Just what ideas she did receive, it is
impossible for us to know, and also the cause of the
excitement she manifested when told about them. At
noon there was to be a launch from a ship-yard near by,
and we seated ourselves near a window, that I might
tell her all I could see. She listened eagerly to the
description of the ship, its position, etc., what the men
were doing, and was much *disappointed* when told that
it would not move, and now they must wait till the water
was higher to launch it. She had learned this word
to-day, and it was a very good occasion on which to use
it. She asked, " Why does God not launch it?"

June 13 She told me she wished to talk about her
teachers, and occupied the hour with reminiscences of all
who had ever taught her anything, what they did, and
even expressed her opinion of how they did it. In talking of her experiences with me, she asked, "Were not
Doctor and J. wrong not to let me come and see you,
and stay with you all the time, when you were sick last
summer? If you are sick again I must come, and I can
stay with you and take care of you, because you teach
me, and I can be still." This occasional assertion o
her rights, and the development of the feeling of respon

sibility, show us how fast the time is approaching when she will put off the little child.

Another topic of conversation was suggested by the question, " Where do men get water to drink? " She asked, in jest, if I would teach her 300 trillions of years. I held up my hands to express surprise, and said, " Yes." She often begins with a joke, but as soon as I answer in the same way. she seems to forget, and takes it all as in earnest. She said now, " Do you play? Will you live so many years?" On the map she completed New Jersey and crossed the Delaware to find Philadelphia, which she has desired to do for a long time, because she has heard so much about it as my home. It seems to be best to have points of interest just ahead of her studies in geography, instead of showing her all such as soon as she takes the map.

June 15. She has learned to do plain sewing very neatly, and always assists in making her own clothes. She threads the needle by feeling the eye with her tongue, and by a rolling motion conducting the thread into it, as most of the blind do. It is some time since she had any sewing, and fearing she might forget to work well, I told her she might do some for me, when she had finished her knitting. " For money?" she asked. " My sister works for me because she wants to oblige me and to help me." "1 am very, very poor, and want money." " What can you buy with money? " She could not think of anything she wanted, but said, " All people have money, Lizzie B." (a little girl) " has money." Told her that her father gave Dr. Howe money to buy her clothes, and it was better for him to take care of it

8

for her. She was more willing to work, but not quite as cheerful about it as I should like to see her.

June 20. She complained of her eyes, which often give her trouble saying, " My eyes are unstrong." When doing her sums she looked troubled, and I said, " I must get a flat-iron to smooth your face." She laughed and asked, " Is it twisted or wrinkled? Are wrinkled and tumbled the same, and jammed and tumbled ? "

While talking of the various kinds of wood, she went from room to room feeling of different articles, and seldom made a mistake between pine, oak, and mahogany. She was puzzled when feeling of a secretary which was veneered, noticed the difference at once, and asked an explanation. She remembered a lesson more than a year ago on the various kinds of trees, and said that men cut down the trees to make the boards. When asked how they knew which tree to cut to make pine or mahogany, she answered, " I think they guess." Described to her the difference in the leaves, bark, etc.

June 21. A question in the arithmetic lesson puzzled her to-day, and we spent an hour upon it, but did not succeed in answering it. " If two men do a piece of work in six days, how long would it take four men to do the same? " This was not a surprise to me, for the child who performs examples of this kind without difficulty at first is a rare exception.

June 22. For some time it has been very irksome to her to write specimens enough to satisfy the demands of visitors, and of late this unwillingness has extended to recitations in geography. This was so manifest when company was present yesterday, that it seemed best to discuss the matter, and put it before her as a duty. The argument that had the most effect was that the blind girls always did as they were asked to by strangers, and that if she did not, they would think she could not learn as well as they. In her writing lesson she was asked to prepare a very nice specimen; and to give more interest in it, I suggested that she write a composition on the camel. This was new, as her writing previously has been either in the form of journal entries or letters. She had been much interested in a talk about camels, deserts, etc., and so wrote as follows, in a very distinct hand: "The camel can go a very long time without drinking; he can carry very heavy loads; he is very gentle like a dove; he goes on very sandy ground; he carries people on his back to ride long."

She suffers much from the heat, and is so listless and dull that only conversations upon animals seem to interest her in such weather as this. Our subject was lions, and she closed a long discussion by saying, "I think men could teach them to be very gentle like sheep."

June 30. A man with a very tame monkey came to the house, and Laura was persuaded to put her hand upon it, and having overcome her first dread she was quite brave and enjoyed feeling of him as he performed his tricks. She had many questions to ask after he had gone, especially as to the manner of teaching monkeys. "Do ourang-outangs learn to do such things? Why do monkeys wear chains? His toes were very long, why? When I gave him a fig he took off his hat to thank me:

he did not know that I could not see." She has, after three lessons, mastered the difficulty in the question on work in arithmetic.

July 3. She performed thirty examples this morning, but is much troubled by the mosquitoes. " I think mosquitoes were very hungry," she said. " Why did God make mosquitoes to bite us? Was He wrong?" A cold wind was blowing, and she asked if the camels in the menagerie in Boston would not have very cold feet, because when they were at home they were always in hot sand.

She knew that the children were planning for a holiday to-morrow, and asked, " Do they call it Fast?" Told her the programme for the celebration of the Fourth of July, and that she might go with me to the grove. This was a new word.

July 5. She seemed to enjoy the day yesterday as much as any one. I told her, as she sat beside me, what was being done, and while we were listening to the oration and poem, both of which were by blind young men, she was very quiet. While going to church she has learned to be perfectly still. I found her in a great frolic with her doll this morning, and helped her to carry it out for a while, but the promised visit to the menagerie soon put everything else out of her mind, and she asked questions about the animals continually.

July 6. We spent four hours in the menagerie. The keeper of the animals was very kind, and, to my surprise, Laura was very calm. She felt of the foot, tusks, and trunk of the elephant and fed him, and examined the saddle. The keeper showed her a young leopard which is yet tame, also a cockatoo. Then I led her from cage to cage, telling what animals were in each, describing their nature, size, and appearance. After this she asked for the monkeys, and we stood beside their cages a long time, while I told her all the tricks they were doing. She frequently laughed aloud. We were disappointed in not having a ride on the elephant, but the crowd began to gather, and as Laura was as much an object of interest to them as the animals, we made good a retreat.

July 7. A rehearsal of the menagerie visit. She wished to talk of the various sizes of the animals, and seemed to be classifying them in her own mind accordingly. In her geography lesson she learned the rivers of Georgia, but thought they were very hard, and that she should not remember them.

July 8. She did such sums as "Thirty is three tenths of what number?" very well, but is unwilling to give the explanation, her excuse being, "It is very long, and I am too weak, and it is very hard for me." Most children, I find, object in like manner. She has been for some weeks unusually quiet, rarely making bad noises, and in their stead we hear her happy, ringing laugh. She has been very patient in the difficulties of arithmetic, and these generally are the greatest trials she has in her studies. She is unwilling to be helped over them, but is determined to conquer them herself, and thus a mental conflict arises, which is very likely to show itself in irritability, extending sometimes to other things, especially if she has to leave her work unfinished at the expiration of the lesson hour.

July 11. While talking she stopped suddenly and said, "Something moves in my side; it is like quicksilver." She had been shown some yesterday, and played with it on a plate. When in her geography, I spelled " Mississippi" to her, she said, " I think it is a very silly name so many doubles and *i s* in it." She did not approve of the word " Alabama" either.

July 12. Laura wanted me to walk to Boston with her, and as I had been ill I told her I must ask Doctor F. if I might go out. That I should be under the direction of any one seemed to be a new thought to her, and she followed it out by questions to see if dis-obedience in my case would lead to similar results as in her own. "What would you do if he said no, but you did not mind him and went? Would you be wrong and silly and deceive him? Would you cry? Could you talk with me when you were very wrong, and where would you stay alone?" In geography she was much amused at finding Providence Island on the coast of Florida, remembering that Providence city is in Rhode Island.

July 14. For a week Laura had had a visit to her former teacher, Mrs. Morton, in prospect, and this morn-ing she surprised me by showing me how she had been spending her spare moments. I found that she had ooked over all her clothes very carefully to see that everything was in order, and had exercised much in-genuity in repairing the old ones. This being done, she wished to do the same for me.

July 15. She had a sum about a pole which was partly under water, etc., and her old difficulty came up again. I supposed she understood it long ago. " Did the man see the pole? Did he think of it?" (with her usual gesture of rapping her forehead.) " Is this a story?" The explanation of the difference between a sum and a story occupied a long time.

July 17. One of the blind girls died last week, and we thought it best to say nothing to Laura about it, but some of the family spoke of it to her, and she met me this morning saying, "Betsy is dead. Why did she die?" " She was very sick." " Where?" " In throat and lungs." " And God was ready for her?" Did Betsy try to breathe again? Why did you not tell me last Wednesday?" " I thought it would make you sad to know she was so sick." " Why did Doctor want to tell me about Orrin, because he wanted to teach me and make me know better?" She remembers that Doctor wished to teach her himself, and so has asked me few questions. She has not been as much excited as she was at the time of Orrin's death.

In geography we have had an entirely new experience. I never knew her to require to be told any names more than twice since she began the study, but this morning I had to tell the rivers and towns in Tennessee and Kentucky for the third time. What there is peculiar in them I cannot see. Reviewed her on the Eastern, Middle, and Southern States, and she did remarkably well, showing that it was caused by no fatigue of mind.

CHAPTER X.

July 18. Our journey to Halifax, Mass., took nearly all the day, as we were obliged to wait a long time for a stage at Stoughton. Laura was very quiet, and worked industriously while we waited. She was much amused at our *tête-à-tête* dinner at the hotel. She asked what the waitress said to me. Told her she asked if we wanted anything. This happened to be a new form of expression, and must be explained. " Did you tell her yes or no ? " " No." After this she perceived that I had some pudding brought me, and a question of my veracity was raised, which took most of the afternoon to settle. When we stopped to water the horses she asked, " Do both horses put their heads in one pail ? How does he know when they want water ? If he hold water and make horses put their heads down, do they not have to drink when they do not want water ? "

It may seem to those accustomed to teach children with all their senses, who acquire knowledge of such things intuitively, that these questions would be tedious to answer, but in justice to my pupil I must say that I doubt if any teacher ever had a work of such interest, and although its very intensity drew heavily upon the nervous energy, yet there could never arise a feeling of impatience at questions so earnestly asked.

The pleasure of teaching was equal to that of being taught, and the reply could always be given, with truth, to the remark so frequently made by visitors, "How much patience it must take to teach her," "Not more than to teach others."

July 19, Halifax. Laura's happiness is so great this morning that she does not know what to do to express it. She remembers the places of things she has seen here before, and leads me to closets where they are, to ask about them. She knows that now she can understand better than when here a year or more ago. A collection of shells interests her much. She enjoys the smoothness of some artifically polished, and the strange shapes of others, and when shown one very thin, she said, " I think the fish liked to keep cool." Her only trouble seems to be to know, " Why did God make troublesome mosquitoes?" Gave her a lesson in the woods, and showed her how men could distinguish between oak and pine. Some time ago she said she thought they guessed, but she soon learned now, so she could tell each tree. Showed her the different kinds of pine, and the cone containing seeds. She wished to feel every tree, and expressed great surprise when told that I could see everywhere around nothing but trees.

July 20. Another lesson on shells; among them found a snake-skin, and this opened an entirely new subject to her. In the woods gave a lesson on the different parts of a tree. Showed her a beech-tree; she admired the leaf very much, and asked, " Why did

you not show it to me yesterday?" It pleased her
when I had to confess it was because I did not know it
myself yesterday. When told a dog was sick, she
asked Mrs. M., "How can you know when a dog is
sick?" "Just as I know when you are sick." "Do
dogs look pale?" When she had forgotten something
she said, "I am very forgetful; my thoughts waste."

July 21. She had some more examples in arithmetic
about work, and found very little difficulty in them.

July 22. Finished the sixth section, and commenced
on miscellaneous examples, which, she says, "I think
are very hard for me."

In this opinion she entirely agrees with a little pupil
whom I taught some years later, who said that all were
very easy "except the questions that lady asks, Mis—
Cellaneous."

A lesson in the barn taught her many new words,
"rake, hoe, axe, saw," etc. She asked me to show
her "the horses' things, bits and shaders" (meaning
blinders). She had learned about these in the stable
at home. She enjoys gathering cherries.

July 24. She was much pleased to examine the
horse with the side-saddle, and to feel the process of
mounting for a ride, my position on the horse, manner
of holding the reins and whip. On my return she asked
questions about the ride, etc., for an hour. She has all
her lessons as when at home, and the good effects of
change of air and scene are visible in her great buoyancy of spirit.

July 26. To a question in arithmetic she answered,
"Fourteen sheeps," and when corrected, said, "No, it
is one sheep, two sheeps." I think she is unwillingly

convinced of her error, and will probably contest the point again. Took her to a place where materials for building a house were collected. She learned about boards, shingles, laths, etc. A little farther on found some trees which had been sawn into planks and piled as they were cut, which gave her a very correct idea of how we get planks and boards. A favorite amusement when we are walking is to ask me, " What do you see?" stopping and holding my hand to give me time to look, and if she thinks I do not give her objects enough she says, " Look more." We spent two hours in this way this morning, stopping to show her every-thing new, and had a very profitable lesson, and a walk of six miles. She wanted to ask if C. and L., two little boys in the family, were alike, and said, " Are they alike, I mean in body?" and then moved her hand over her face. 1 asked if she wanted to know if they looked alike. " Yes." Told her they were very unlike. " How do you know they are unlike?" "Are their hands alike?" " No; L.'s are soft and fat, but C.'s are tough and rough." Talking of mosquitoes she said, fretfully, " I do not want them to touch me again " I replied, " You can ask them to please to let you alone." " And what shall we do if they do not mind?" She then raised a question about our right to kill them, which I settled by telling her that we could not talk to them and tell them it was wrong to trouble us, and so killed them.

July 28. An order for specimens of writing obliged us to take time from other lessons to attend to it. One, which I thought very good, read as follows: " I went to Boston with Oliver & very many folks, to see the

caravan. In the tent I saw the elephant's tusks, &
legs, & trunk, & foot; his skin was very rough. I gave
him a very great many pieces of apple. I put them in
his trunk, he moved it to take them, and put in his
mouth. We went into the saddle; then I saw a very
pretty parrot, & a very gentle leopard — he was very
little and pretty."

July 29. Reviewed the lessons of the week, and
when talking of the trees she brought a pine cone to
ask why it had opened so much since she brought it
into the house. When told it was dying, she said, '' It is
dead. Can God make it grow again?" Explained to
her how the seeds fell into the ground and then the
trees grew up from them, and other cones grew with
more seeds, but this old cone was good for nothing and
thrown away. At dinner she moved her hand through
the air, and asked, '' When we do so, do we cut the
air?" Talked about ribbon, and asked if she knew of
what it was made. More than a year ago she had
learned something about it. She replied, '' Silk." '' On
what does silk grow?" '' The silk-worm makes it."
'' Do you think the silk-worm makes the ribbon?"
'' No." She told me about '' the ball" the silk-worm
made to wind his silk upon, and asked, '' Why do they
have very, very nice cotton-wool?" She looked much
troubled when she found her feeling had deceived her,
and that it was silk, not cotton, and said sadly, '' I
think I could not know by feeling."

Aug. 3. Lesson to-day was multiplication of numbers from twelve to twenty, mentally, which she performed readily. In her hour for conversation she asked
why there was so much work about the room. It

belonged to a company of ladies who were assisting the Fall River sufferers, and I thought it a good opportunity to give her a lesson on it. Told her how much the fire burned, and then of the poor people who had no home or clothes. She seemed unable to understand its full extent, for she said, " The fire did not burn the chambers?" When told what the ladies were sewing, and how kind they were to assist the poor people, she said, " I think the men must go out in the woods where 1 was with you, that are very thick, and cut much wood, and send to the poor people, because they will be very cold when it is cold weather. What will they do before they have more houses?" In geography she has completed the States, the boundaries, capitals, rivers, and towns; now I shall go over them again, teaching her the productions, climate, objects of interest, etc. The last lesson of the day was given in the stage-coach, on the subject of horses. She always asks their color, name, disposition, and many other particulars. In reply to some trivial question, I replied, " I do not know." She said, " God knows, we can ask him when we go to him." She was feeling very sad in leaving Halifax and her dear friend Mrs. Morton.

Aug. 5. Completed the seventh section of Colburn's Mental Arithmetic.

Aug. 8. The blind children were all going on a berrying excursion, and no one was to be left at home. So 1 offered my services as housekeeper, thinking I could make it quite as profitable to Laura as a regular lesson would be. After breakfast told her we must wash the dishes, and she went to assist me very willingly. During the day she had many opportunities for usefulness, and the day with its unusual lessons was not a lost one.

Aug. 9. Forty sums in reducing mixed numbers to improper fractions. Told her a story about the way the elephants crossed Bristol Ferry; one went in a boat, but the other, refusing to obey orders, swam across. She talked an hour about it; asked if the elephants touched the ground under the water, and when told they swam on top of it, she asked, "How can elephants go so, when they are very large and heavy? Do not steamboats touch the ground when they are heavy?" Next came questions like these: "If the elephants would not mind, were they wrong?" She had noticed the children had bad coughs, and was told the name "whooping-cough," but did not believe it could come if they had not taken cold. Sitting beside me one day she perceived I held my breath for a long time, and was very much frightened, and said, "Did you almost die? Your breath stopped." She is very fond of playing the nurse, and has many suggestions of remedies to make. One day, after exercising in the gymnasuim, she found that my hands were hot and swollen. Her sympathies were much excited. She brought a silver pencil-case. bottle, key, and everything cold that she could think of for me to hold. Then a bright thought struck her, and she led me to an iron-bound trunk, saying, "If you put your hands on this, I think you will be better." A lesson on commerce, which was a new subject.

Aug. 11. Reducing improper fractions to mixed numbers gave her some trouble.

When she has been called in the morning lately, we

have found her dressing. Asked her how she knew when to get up. " I put my hand on the door to feel it shake." " Do you get up to go to the door?" " No, the door that is by my bed. I put my finger in the key-hole, and if the girls are up it shakes. Who jumps and slams the door in the morning? Why do girls open and shut doors in the night?"

Her own room was in a remote corner of the house, quite removed from the other sleeping-rooms, and we should hardly perceive with our ears the noises which she speaks of feeling.

Aug. 12. She overcame the difficulties in her arithmetic and said, " I think I was very dull not to know before." She has had a lesson on the use of the period. To show how many lessons will be required before she can be taught to punctuate properly. we give below her account of a story which was read to her yesterday, with her punctuation : —

" Little George's mother is very poor. instead of having bright coalfires. she has dry sticks to burn. So she sent George two miles. to try to get as much woods as he could. After he had done work very hard. the sun was high over his head   he was hot and tired and hungry. he wanted some dinner. so he had bread and butter. he went to find cool place. and found a stone with green moss by the brook. then he went to look for very large leaf to dip off the water. His stone was his table. he sat on bank. brook was his wine-cellar. Then he heard birds sing very loudly in the trees. He went to pick some wild red strawberries. and put leaf in his cap to keep them nice. he thought that they were very ripe and good. he wanted half but he thought that he would save many berries. When it was dark then he went home. then his mother called him to come. he ran and put the woods in her washhouse. Then he gave her some berries and she said 'did he save them for his sick mother? to make her better?' she was very glad. he felt very happy to have her eat them."

Aug. 14. Laura completed to-day the eighth section in arithmetic, in five months from the time she commenced the book. The word "merrily" was the first topic of conversation, and then she wished to know if we said "more, morest," and "much, muchest," and why not? Used the word "complain," supposing she understood it, but found it was a new word.

Aug. 15. Her lesson was multiplying fractions and reducing the result to a mixed number. She surprised me by doing the examples without any trouble. While at work with her types, she wiped her eyes several times, at last she said, "My eyes are very vexatious this morning." This is a word she has lately learned; it pleases her much, so she uses it on many occasions. A lady visited the school who wore unusually thickly lined sleeves; this she noticed at once and said, "The lady must live in Africa, and then she will not have to wear such thick clothes." At three o'clock this morning Laura was found playing with her cups and saucers. When I asked her why she got up in the night to play, she said, "Jennie is sick, and I was giving her medicines." She carries out a play with a doll further than I ever knew any other child. Everything she has ever known done for a sick person is tried upon the doll. She is moved from one bed to another and as carefully bolstered up as if she were a child.

Aug. 18. We talked about Indians, their manner of living, wigwams, color. She asked about the people of Africa, and when told they were black asked, " Why did God make some people black?" Told her they lived in Boston before the white people came from England, and their name for it. She enjoys a lesson on such a subject, it gives her so many new ideas. A question in geography, which I asked without a thought of puzzling her, occupied most of the hour in the explanation : " Which of the New England States has no sea-coast?"

Tried the experiment of reading " The Spider and the Fly " to her. Transposed some of it into prose and read very slowly, explaining such words as she might not understand, and told her it was a story in which the man who wrote it played that the spider and the fly could speak. She was amused at the idea and retained it some time, but at last, with a look of surprise, said, " *Did* fly *say* so?" It seemed to me that she understood it, but the proof will be to-morrow.

Aug. 19. She failed entirely in telling the story of yesterday.

Aug. 21. Read it to her very carefully again, and asked her to tell it to me. She makes a strange mixture of conversational and narrative style, but gets a pretty good idea of it. She has found a toy horse, and taken her doll from bed to have her take a ride, saying, very seriously, " I think she will be much better, for riding horseback will make her strong." She had a very important question to ask, " Do the negroes wash their hands? Because black does not get dirty very quick, and I thought they need not wash their hands very often."

13

Aug. 23. Tenth section. She was a little puzzled at first, but I gave her some cards to cut to illustrate the principle, and she did twenty-five examples. Talked with her about Niagara Falls. When I told her about them some months ago, she understood that the stones fell constantly with the water. When told of the roaring noise they made, she said, " Can you hear it? Try and see." Mrs. W., her friend, is in Saratoga, and she asked, " Can she hear them? Can my mother in Hanover hear them? Why did not Dr. Howe go to hear them? Why did not he tell me about them?" " Because when he went away you did not know about many places, and could not have understood what he said if he had tried to tell you, but when he comes home you can ask him." She looked much surprised and said, " He will be very busy writing very much and he cannot talk, and he will not be in this school-room so I cannot ask him." Told her she could ask him as well in the study as in the school-room ; but she seemed to think it would be necessary for him to have the map before him in order to talk about the Falls.

Aug. 24. In a section in arithmetic which generally puzzles children, she did forty sums such as " One third of two is how many thirds of one? " She was doubtful about the difference between "better" and "best." As she had used them a long time. I supposed she understood them perfectly. She told me, " J. says if I am gentle and good, Mrs. Howe will send me a doll with a strange kind of a dress ; you will not know about it." When talking about its name, she thought she should call it Miss Dewey, but after a moment's thought said, " No, doll must be Julia Ward."

Aug. 27. She brought " The Child's Second Book " and asked me to explain " possess," " general description," and lastly the plate of the Solar System, at the end of the book. Here was a work indeed for me to begin upon, but after reflection I decided that she could be told much that would be both interesting and profitable to her. Commenced by telling her the great distance of the sun from us, of its size. " Can we go there? " was her first question. Asked her how she thought we could go. " In boats." " Do you think there is water all the way to the sun? " " No, go in cars." " Is there land? " " No," and pointing to the sun she said, "It is air," and was puzzled to know what we could do. I hoped she would suggest a balloon, as 1 had given her a lesson upon them, but she evidently did not understand much about them, and so they did not occur to her. " Can flies go up to the sun? Can God be at the sun? " She was anxious for me to begin the explanation of the plate, but 1 told her, before she was ready for that, I must tell her of many things. Talked of the size of the stars, how large they appeared to us. The idea that distance made objects look smaller was new to her, and she was filled with wonder when, to exemplify it, I told her if I were to sit in my room and see her, walking to the Point, she would grow smaller, and would, when there, look like a very little girl. From this, she could understand why the moon should look so much larger than the sun because so much nearer; told her of the planets, their names, and on which we lived; she asked what the lines were for on the plate. Forgetting that

she was just receiving her first idea, I made too long a
step and said they were to show where the planets
moved round the sun, and that it took the earth three
hundred and sixty-five days, so we called it a year. She
said, " I think then Louisa's father" (a sea captain)
" went to the sun, he is gone three years." This showed
how little she appreciated what had been said. When
she found I had been teaching her astronomy she said,
" Will you please write and tell Doctor what I study?"

Aug. 29. She was impatient to resume the subject
of yesterday. " Are there people in the sun?" When
told we could not know, she said, " We can ask God
when we go to heaven." " Can I see when I go to
heaven, to see the sun?" Talked about the motions of
the earth. When she learned that it was turning round
all the time, she said, " When I am dizzy then I feel the
floor go round." To explain the cause of day and
night, I put a pin into a ball of yarn to represent
Boston, supposed the fire in the grate to represent the
sun, and by revolving the ball let her see that one side
must be in the dark. She seemed to understand this.

Aug. 31. The lesson was upon the difference in time
between places, illustrated by a second pin to represent
London. She soon learned to tell what the time was
in the one, having it given in the other. In her geography lesson, and when apparently very happy, she
took both hands from the map, and with a look of
despair said, " Are you not very tired of living so many
years?" " No, are you?" " Yes, I want to go to God
in heaven." Some time ago the same thought came to
her under similar circumstances. It seems to me that
she gets a momentary glimpse of the field of knowl-

edge to be explored, and its immensity overwhelms her.

Sept 1. She was in much trouble in her arithmetic, because of another sum about work. The old difficulty, which I thought overcome long ago, arose, and she could not tell how long it would take one man to do a piece of work if it took three men twenty-one days.

Sept. 4. For some time we have noticed some little developments in Laura which looked like prudery. On Saturday evening, at the children's party held in the Doctor's parlors, Dr. Lieber attempted to shake hands with her. She pulled her hand away, and refused to speak to him at all, or to any one standing near her. There was a little excuse for her; there had been a great crowd at the exhibition in the afternoon, she had become much excited, and the heat had made her head ache, but the time had come to treat the matter seriously, and this morning we discussed it. She talked of the different times when she had acted rudely, showing she was perfectly conscious to what I alluded. When told how ladies and other blind girls behaved, she confessed that she had been silly, and promised she would never do so again. She asked the meaning of " prevent " and " explanation." Some time since she had had the word " description," and now asked, " Did you give me a *description* of the new word prevent, or an *explanation* of it?" She shows much ingenuity in introducing these long words into her conversation, but not unfrequently I find she has not taken their exact meaning. Ater a long talk about the caves of Virginia, she gave me a kiss and hug, and said, " You are very kind to give me many descriptions."

Sept. 8. She reminded me of a promise to show her a tellurian. She very readily told me from it about day and night, and the time at the different quarters of the globe, but found it hard to realize that some people were then sleeping. She noticed at once the revolution of the earth on its own axis, and also about the sun, and in good language told the effects produced by each motion.

Sept. 9. From week to week I can see an improvement in her way of repeating the stories which are read to her, and to-day she did better than ever before. When she writes one out fully, there are many mistakes in the use of language, which never occur when she is spelling it out with the fingers; but this is readily accounted for when we remember that writing is of necessity a slow process, and that she cannot look back to read her last sentence, or to note the omission of a word by inadvertence.

CHAPTER XI.

PERHAPS some reader would like to ask, " How
do you read books to Laura?" Seated at her left
side, on a sofa rather than in a chair, with the book
in my left hand I spell with my right hand (using
the manual alphabet of the deaf-mutes) every
word with the exception of "and," which has its
own sign. This is all I have to attend to. She
takes care of the rest herself. With her right
hand moving lightly over my fingers, never with
pressure enough to impede their motion, she
spells or rather reads the words. She does not
seem to take cognizance of each letter any more
than we do when we read with our eyes, but the
most rapid talker by the finger alphabet could
never be too quick for her comprehension, and I
always talk to her with such rapidity that no eye
could possibly read the words. Constant practice (and for a year I had talked more with my
fingers than with my mouth) had made them very
flexible, and the question was so often asked me,
"How fast do you talk?" that I carefully tried
some experiments, which resulted as follows: If a

person seated near me read aloud, I could not interpret as rapidly as she read, but if she was reading to a number of people in a large room, I could follow her, giving Laura every word spelled upon my fingers. Of course the mere spelling was no more an act of consciousness than it is when we are writing; no one thinks how he spells his words, unless in doubt of the orthography, so that no time was lost in this way.

Sept. 12. The constant rubbing had caused Laura's hands to be very rough. Dr. Fisher noticed them, and told her she must put some ointment upon them and wear gloves. This was a great trial, for it not only retarded her own talking, but made it difficult for her to understand me. She tried to be patient, and after a day or two succeeded in using them despite the gloves. In her lesson on the tellurian she learned about the length of the year on the different planets, and of her own accord, entered upon a calculation of how old she would be if she had lived in the others. Herschel amused her, and she had a hearty laugh when she found how few years old Dr. H. would be had he lived there.

Sept. 13. The questions which she solved readily this morning were of this kind: "If five eighths of a cask of wine cost forty-two dollars, what will the whole cost?" She answered nine such in her lesson of three quarters of an hour and explained them.

Among our visitors to-day were two gentlemen who had walked from North Carolina. Laura's knowledge of the States they had passed through furnished many topics for conversation. When she asked about Wier's

Cave, one of them presented her with a piece of a stalactite which he had brought from it. This morning when she came for her lesson, she asked if I could see the sun ; told her I could, but it was not high enough yet for her to feel it. A while after she said, "I think the earth moves round very slowly, I cannot feel the sun much." She enjoyed examining the planetarium, and spent an hour over it.

Sept. 15. Her doll in Welsh costume arrived last evening, and furnished a topic for conversation. She wished to know about the people and their country. She told me that her old doll and Julia (the new one) loved each other very much.

Sept. 21. Our lesson was on merchant ships, suggested by her inquiry, " What does Mr. W. do in Boston all day ? " Described the preparations for the voyage, loading the ship, and then of the return cargo. Her last question was, " Where does he get money to buy so many things? "

Sept. 25. A little circumstance occurred at the teatable last eve which troubled me. She had eaten one piece of pie and asking for another, was told it was not best for her to eat more. She was displeased, and sat still until she thought I had left the room, when she asked Mrs. S. for it. As this savored of both deception and disobedience, I talked seriously about it this morning. She confessed at once the error; but justified herself saying, " I wanted more pie." Found Mrs. Smith had promised her the pie for lunch to-day and decided it was best to let her have it, that she must give part of it to Frank and Susan (two little deaf-mute children) who wanted it as much as she did, and did not ask for it after their teacher had told them no. She did not object to this, but said, " I will give you some too." Told her I only wished to teach her to do right, not to take her pie. She said, " It is to remember me that I must not do so again, and next time when you tell me that I must not have any more, I shall not ask Smith for it." She is reviewing the boundaries of the States; she does not enjoy it, and when I proposed it, said, " I have told you many times, I *know*."

Sept. 29. The day was spent in reviews, and arrangements for the vacation. She objected to my proposal that she write an hour every day in her journal during my absence, but consented to it at last, that I might have the pleasure of seeing it on my return. Of course she must miss her lessons, but she bade me good by saying, " I am glad for you to go and see your friends, because it will make you very happy." One day in the vacation she had the promise of going to meet her mother in Halifax, but a violent rain prevented. She said, "God was very unkind to make it rain, he knew we wanted to go." She was reconciled by being told that the earth needed rain to make the things grow, and she must try to be happy when disappointed.

Oct. 27. She asked why Mercury and Venus had no moons. When told we did not know, she said, " We can ask God about it when we go to heaven. Does Orrin* know about it now?" Thought she might have forgotten some of her geography lessons in the month, and gave her a review. She answered questions as fast as her fingers could fly, and made only four mistakes in

---

* The little blind boy who died two years ago.

all the States. She mentioned all the capitals and on what rivers situated.

Nov. 1. Before breakfast I went to get seed for the birds, but could not find the glass with which I measured it, which always stood on a waiter. At the table I asked Laura if she knew where it was. She answered without hesitation, " I have not seen it." On searching for it further, I was surprised to find it on the floor in a corner, broken in pieces, as if it had been thrown with considerable force. A suspicion that all was not right with Laura, led me to watch her countenance while she was doing her morning work. After school I asked again, " Do you know where the glass is?" The blood rushed to her face, and she said hesitatingly. " I thought you let something fall yesterday, when I was in the kitchen knitting." From this reply I knew she was guilty, and said, " Think, — be sure to tell the truth." Then she said, " When I went down yesterday, I saw the flies eating crumbs in the waiter, and I brushed them away, flies were eating glass, and I did not want them to, and I thought I felt glass fall." " But you said before you thought that *I* let something fall. Did I break the glass?" " No." " Where did the glass fall?" "On the floor." " Did you feel it there?" " Yes." " Why did you not tell me when I asked this morning? I looked for it, but it was so dark I could not see the pieces on the floor." She repeated what she had said before, but in a very indifferent and careless manner, and it seemed to me with a disposition to " brave it out," which was an entirely new development and gave me great anxiety.

Penitence has followed always so quickly after transgression, that it almost made us feel that her faults were so little we ought to let them pass unnoticed. I told her now, I could not talk any more about it, but that she must sit alone, without work, and think about it. Without her knowledge, I stayed in the room, where I could carefully watch her. In a little while her countenance changed, and she became troubled, and soon the tears fell. At the close of the forenoon I went to her, and asked, "Why do you think you are sitting alone?" "To think about being wrong, and deceiving you. At table I said I had not seen, and at nine, I said I frightened flies away; it was not true." She asked why I did not cry as she did. Told her I felt very sad, and it would be long before I could be happy, and that Doctor would be very sad when he read in my journal about it. "Did I act a lie, or tell a lie?" she asked. I talked with her some time, to try to convince her how much better it would have been had she come and told me at once after she had done it. She said, "I talked to myself about its being a lie, and that it was wrong to deceive." After sitting still awhile, with the tears rolling down her cheeks, she said, "My mother told me I would (should) be a good girl. I hope I shall learn to tell the truth, and always to tell you and Miss J., when I do anything. Are you tired of teaching me not to tell a lie?" Told her I hoped she would learn soon that it was much pleasanter and easier to tell the truth, and that she might remember this very ong, she had better sit alone to work. "Will you shut the door that no one can come in, and see a very sad and wrong little girl?" After an hour I went for her to walk. She seemed glad to go, but talked little. On returning, she went to the school-room to see com-

pany, it being trustees' meeting. After this she said,
" I had better sit alone till tea-time." At the tea-table
she said, " I want to tell you something. Miss M——
is here to see Lurena to-day : may I go to see her?"
Asked her if she thought it would be right for me to let
her go. In a moment she said, " No, I must sit alone
to-night, and think about being wrong." When going to
bed she said, " Will you forgive me?" and with a very
sad look, " Do you think I will ever tell lies again?"
I have noted this case so carefully because it is the
first untruth since the affair of the gloves that we have
known of. There is no reason why she should not have
told me of the accident at once, for she had seemed to
take pleasure previously in doing so, and has never
been reproved for any such thing.

Nov. 2. She recited an excellent lesson in arithmetic, and never seemed to love me so well as to-day.
Gave her a lesson on the large map of North America.
She has been studying on a map of the United States,
and the scale of the new one was of course very different. To give her an idea of this, I passed her hand
over the space occupied by the United States. It rested
on Missouri, which she spelled. 1 asked her to find
Ohio, not thinking it possible for her to do it without
help, but she had no difficulty, and told me some of the
rivers and capitals. I supposed we should have two
lessons, at least, on the United States, before beginning
the other countries of North America, but it was all
lone in this one. When I showed her the little space
occupied by the Gulf of Mexico, she immediately
showed me Florida. At each school to-day she asked,
" Do you feel more happy? I must try to be very

good, to make you more happy. If I say my lesson well, will it make you happy?"

Nov. 3. In learning about Mexico and Guatemala, she said, "I think there are many new hard names." Why one name should be any harder than another to her, has been a question that I have tried in vain to answer satisfactorily to myself. If we see or hear an unusual combination of letters, we call it "a hard word," but neither of these causes operate with her, nor does she always classify words as we should, for sometimes a word which seems simple to me, gives her difficulty. Some one had told her that bears sometimes ate little boys. I explained it, and she said, "Bears are not to blame." "Why?" "Because they are hungry and have a good appetite." She asked if all animals were ferocious (a new word to-day). She saw at the menagerie a little leopard three months old, and very gentle, but I told her it would become wild as it grew older. "Who takes care of the young leopard, that other animals might not eat him? Why does God make some animals wild?"

Nov. 6. At noon she came to me saying, "I found some words in a book I do not know." She attempted to spell one, and I guessed from the rest of the sentence what it was, "Alphabet are twenty-six in number." I supposed she knew the word long ago, for a year or more since, when she was daily using her type box, she used to arrange the letters in proper order, but proba·bly then I always spoke of them to her as the letters. For our talk to-day, told her she might think of all the animals we required to make the different things in the room, and to illustrate my meaning I asked, "What one to make the carpet?" This was sufficient clew, and her thoughts and fingers seemed to fly. "Wool from the sheep, horse to make hair-cloth for chairs and sofa, goat to make the cushion for the other rocking-chair, and baby." "What do you mean by baby?" "Goat's baby to make my shoes, and silk-worm for my shades, and your handkerchief." Here she paused, and I led her to the table. She put her hand on the thermometer, and said elephant for that and paper-folder, bees for the wax flowers and fruit, birds for the lamp, and whales for oil, and whale's head for my rabbit. This was a little model made of spermaceti.

Nov. 7. Continued yesterday's talk, taking up metals. She thought at once of gold for thimbles, rings, and pins, silver for wire and cologne stand. iron for grate and register and brass. Then she walked about the room to see what she could find. There were few things that she did not know. Next she led me to the basement, and opened the ice chest to ask what it was lined with, and then to the kitchen range to know what the plate on which the maker's name was printed was made of, and to a water pipe that was in the corner of an entry, where no one would suppose she would ever have found it, and lastly to the stairs to ask why part of the supports of the railing were of iron and part of wood. I wondered how many children with their eyes had noticed this. Although I have been with her so long she is a constant surprise to me.

Yesterday I obtained some of Abbott's stories to read, for I find no others are so well adapted to her, and now she can learn so much from stories of the right kind.

Nov. 9. She said, "I want to ask you about many

things that I have seen some time, and where they grow." One of these was a pumpkin. She had seen a very large one, and imagined that it grew upon a tree, and was puzzled to know why it did not fall off. We had a talk upon the manner of growth of various vegetables and fruits, their order of ripening, etc.

Nov. 10. Continued the talk about things in the room, what woods we should need to make them. She knew these all except rosewood. Found she knew nothing about glass. Told her about its manufacture, and the manner of its discovery. She could hardly believe me when I told her that a long time ago men did not know anything about it, and had no glass, and this developed an idea which I never knew before that she had, viz., that God taught the first man everything, and he taught everybody else. The idea of invention or discovery was a new one. The making of soap and paint, white lead, more than filled up her hour, and I felt that she had too much that was new to remember it all.

Nov. 13. Found she could tell me all the story about glass, its discovery, and even the name of the city where it was first used; though only told her once. She was very happy in the hour for company to be introduced to some ladies from Santa Cruz, and that she could show them upon the map where their island was. A talk to-day upon colors, what made from, where the plants grow, etc.

Nov. 14. Commenced Section 13, Colburn's Mental Arithmetic. I anticipated difficulty, but after giving her the first example, left her to think about it. She soon solved it, and did fourteen sums. A talk

upon cochineal. Her delight is great when her recently
acquired knowledge comes into use, as when told that
the insects came from Mexico. Commenced Abbott's
story called " Caleb in Town."

Nov. 17. Finished the large map of North America,
and merely for the experiment took her to a little map
of the same, which is in the corner of the large map of
the United States. She found every place I asked her
except Newfoundland. For a talk, took a summary of
things in the room, saying to what kingdom their component parts belonged. She omitted bees, and I
asked her of what the fruit in the vase was made.
" I do not know, God made it." When naming the
metals she said, " Is zinc good for windows?" Some
of the long windows opening upon a piazza had zinc
set in the lower part of the sash to prevent breakage,
and she had supposed we could see through it as well,
but that it was stronger than glass.

Nov. 18. She asked, " What do you do when you
are frightened and feel warm?" " Look to see what
made me frightened." " Why did something make a
noise under my closet floor, so that I could feel it?"
Here she scratched upon the table to show me, and I told
her it was mice running about, and I had heard them.
" Were you much frightened?" " No. I only thought
they were having a play." " Why did I not think so?"
She seems not to overcome this timidity, and it causes
her real suffering. She writes a great many letters for
her own amusement, and entirely without oversight or
any dictation. It often amuses us to observe how
carefully she adapts herself to her correspondents. The
following is a copy of one she brought me to-day to

14

send to a little sister of mine, who she knows is not acquainted with any of the people about her here, so she has only one or two subjects to make up a letter.

MY DEAR LITTLE LIZZIE:

Miss Swift was sick in her head this morning. Before dinner I brushed her head very much, & put much cologne on, & it made her very much better. She said that I was very kind to her, & she thanked me very much for me to cure her, so she went to church once in the afternoon. I love her very much. I am very happy because I was so very kind to her. I send very much love to you & a kiss. I want to see you very much. My mother & father came to see me & staid seven days. I was very glad to see them last October. I like my little sugar bird very much that you sent it to me by Swift.

My friend, good-bye,

MISS LAURA BRIDGMAN.

This signature was a new thought and originated probably in a sense of her superiority to her little correspondent, and the wish to express it

Nov. 20. She brought to-day a book of diagrams belonging to a work on natural philosophy, and as I make it a point never to discourage her by saying she annot understand about anything, I promised to tell her to-morrow, that I might get time to select enough for a lesson to satisfy her cravings for knowledge. I happened to ask the question, " In what direction does the Mississippi *run?*" This was a new expression to her. Probably I have always used the word " flow " before. She said, " The river has no feet, why do you say *run?*" Continued our talks, asking her the places to which we would have to go to get all the things we needed for the parlor.

Nov. 21. She came, saying, "Get the philosophy." Told her I needed no book, and she waited impatiently for me to begin. It was raining violently, and I concluded to take rain, snow, and hail for my topic. I asked her about the steam from a kettle over the fire. At first she seemed to know nothing about it, but suddenly the memory of a burn she got from it when a little girl came to her, and after that she understood it. Next told her of the effect of the sun's heat upon the water on the earth. The first time she got no idea of it, but on repetition she understood it entirely, and gave me a good explanation in her own words. In teaching her any new thing I always pause at intervals, and ask her to tell me what I have been talking about, that I may be sure she has taken my exact idea. If I omit this, by accident, we are sure to have to begin again at the commencement. Having understood about the way the sun produces vapor, it was an easy step to rain and hail. None but those who have attempted it can fully understand the difficulty of commencing a new subject with Laura. I must be very careful that no word is used in the explanation I give which is new to her. For instance: this morning after explaining the word "vapor," I said, "The sun turns water into vapor." Now no one would think there was anything objectionable in this, but she asked, "Do you mean *turns round?*" She had never chanced to have the word used in the sense of *changes*, and all her attention centred on that one word, and the truth I wished to teach her was lost. If this were the case in only one sentence, it would be of no importance, but occurring frequently, despite all my care, it increases the difficulty much. In one of her lessons to-day she seeemed lazy and sleepy. I rapped on her forehead (a sign which she had adopted herself). She said, " Why?" "To see if you have anything in it, have you?" " No, have you?" " Yes, brains." " My brains are asleep. Are brains and thoughts the same? How do people know about brains?"

Nov. 27. Sunday. She said, " I am thinking about God. I want to go to heaven very much. I want to be very good." While taking a walk she returned to the subject, and said, " I was thinking much about God." On returning from church I found she had taken from the bookcase a copy of the Book of Proverbs in raised type. She said, " It is Proverbs' Book," and asked the meaning of a number of words. " Seek first." " Do you think much of heaven? I do." " What is thine?" Being told that it was the same as " yours," she said, " I think thine and possession are the same." She had learned this word when she was taught " British Possessions " on the map of North America.

Nov. 28. Told her Thursday would be a holiday. " Is it Fast?" Gave her the word " Thanksgiving," and said that I was going to spend the day with an aunt. She asked to be allowed to go to the city to meet me on my return, and I agreed to it, if she could find any one to go with her. She said, " Does God know who will take me? Is God ever surprised?" It seems that, without a teacher, she is working out truths regarding God.

Dec. 5. She was asking many questions about J.'s
going to Boston, and how she was to come back.
She told her, "In my own carriage." This puzzled her
much; she asked, "Why cannot I ride too?" "Because
there is not room." She talked a long time, completely
mystified, and then I asked her what horses took her to
Boston yesterday? "My cloak, bonnet, etc." "Did your
head take you?" "No," but still she did not understand
it until I told her the horses' names were Feet, and then
she laughed heartily and asked, "Who is the driver?"
"The head." She held her hands up to her forehead as
if holding reins, and said, "My soul drives," and then
changed it to, "Think drives."

Dec. 6. Her lesson was forty sums in Section 14.
Asked the meaning of "den, lack, cling, instance."
"How do we know that God lives in heaven?"
When told we read it, "How could God talk to
men and tell them what to write in a book?" And
then she made a noise which she calls talking, and
asked if it was in that way. She said, "Dr. Howe
said, he wanted to tell me all about God." At the time
of Dr. Howe's marriage, it was evident that the question often arose in her mind, though never expressed in
words, whether the new relations might not leave less
space for herself in his affections, but this morning,
December 7, it found utterance. "Does Doctor love me
like Julia?" She was answered, "No." "Does he love
God like Julia?" "Yes." When she came for her lesson,
she repeated the question to me, adding, "God was
kind to give him his wife." Noticing, as I had often
done before, that thoughts of this kind, even though
her better nature asserted itself in the end, were apt to

leave her in a state of mind that would readily develop into impatience, I alluded playfully to the manner the cat was washing her face, and this happening to be a new thought, diverted her attention. She could not understand how it was possible for pussy to use her paw without scratching herself, and we had a lesson an hour long on a kitten. At another time she asked if mules were so very sure-footed because they had more toes than other animals, which held in the ground.

Dec. 12. On being shown where she had done wrong in not observing the wishes of Miss J , she said, "I will not do it again. My thoughts tell me when I am good and when I am wrong." Gave her the new word " conscience." She repeated the story that I had read to her yesterday very well, remembering all the new words. Her written abstracts do not compare favorably with the oral ones, for she cannot be made to feel that it is necessary to take time and paper to write fully as she talks, and in attempting abbreviations she makes mistakes.

It is for this reason that her written productions cannot, with justice, be compared with these of the deaf-mutes who can see ; for if she could look over her own papers after writing, she would herself be surprised at the mistakes, and be able to correct most of them without having them pointed out.

Dec. 14. Not in the right mood for arithmetic, therefore it took an hour to do one example, although very easy. A lesson upon various shapes and the names of each had interested her much yesterday, and to-day she had collected in her mind all things in the house which were irregular in shape, to be told new names. In this

way found she did not know the names of the most
common cooking utensils, so the kitchen was our school-
room. This led to a talk on meats. She said, " I
thought turkey and chicken and ducks were all the
same, they taste alike to me. I can tell beef from
mutton, why can I not know turkey and chicken? "

On a previous page allusion is made to the fact that
we thought that an improvement was perceptible in her
sense of smell, and this has continued, though very
gradual. She has always been a sufferer from a severe
catarrhal affection, and as this shows signs of improvement, we hope for a corresponding one in both smell
and taste.

Dec. 15. She asked if the weather was pleasant, and
being told it looked like snow she said, " Is God getting the snow ready to fall now? " As she had recently
had lessons on vapor, rain, hail, and snow, I recalled
them to her by saying that the vapor had come into the
cold air, and it was freezing the clouds now, so they
would fall in snow, which she understood. Her geography lesson was upon Chili, the Argentine Republic,
and Patagonia with adjacent islands, and completed
the map of South America.

Dec. 18. She commenced Section 15, which puzzled her. Yesterday, when out of school, she read
in a history prepared for the blind, and asked me an
explanation of the sentence, " Their arms were successful." I explained the last word and changed the subject. This morning, after she had done one sum, she
said, " My arms were very successful." Told her I
thought it was her head that was successful in thinking
about the sums, endeavoring to correct the false impression she had received.

At some time she must know all the terrible things of history, wars and fightings, their causes and conse- quences, but my heart sank within me when this ques- tion opened the subject, and as I had not the privilege of telling her of the antidote to the sorrows and suffer- ings of this life, I felt justified in leaving the story of its woes.

Dec. 18. While she was sitting at work this after- noon, I noticed that she made a fretting noise continu- ally, and asked, "Why do you fret to-day?" "Some- thing troubles me." "What is it?" "I want to go to heaven; people are not kind to me, and do not love me here as God does." "What people?" "Many people." "What names?" "Rogers and Wight and Coolidge" (all teachers). "Am not I kind to you?" "Yes." "Why do you think they are not?" "Because they never come and sit by me, and talk to me much." Told her they all had much work to do for the other scholars, and could not have time to talk long with her, but they talked when they met her.

She is always anxious to talk with every one, and knows that often persons who pass her in the house avoid her, as they must do when hurrying to some duty. At such times it is not strange that the feeling of being slighted should show itself; indeed, it is a cause of sur- prise to me that this does not lead to expressions which show a painful appreciation of her privations; but in all the years I have been with her I have never known of such, and I do not think she suffers from this cause.

Dec. 19. She led me to the china closet, saying, "I want to ask you about a shape," and handed me a glass with seven sides. She had learned previously "octagon" and "hexagon." Next she found a twelve-sided glass, and then one with five sides, and another with ten. When she had learned all these hard names, and had seated herself to talk, she asked, "How do we know there is air? Why did God give us air? What is wind made of? Orrin's breath went away when he died. Why do we have blood? If we tie up our wrist very tight. so that blood cannot run, what will our hand do?" In geography she learned for the first time about a volcano. Her questions were numerous : "When did the fire begin to come out? Who made the fire? Is it like the fire in our stoves? Can people go up on a volcano, will it burn them?" Then she thought of Niagara, and asked, "How steep does the water fall? Why does it not stop? Will it never stop? Why does it make a loud noise? Is it like a cannon?"

The gradual development of her mind is shown very clearly in this way ; when first told about a new thing, Niagara for instance, she asks all the questions which occur to her at that time, but after a few months more of study, her field of inquiry is enlarged, and then she returns voluntarily to the subject for more information.

Finding one of the canary birds dead, thought it a good time to let her examine it, as she has often tried to do when held in my hand alive. She asked, "Why did it die?" "Are the other birds lonely and sad?" "Why cannot you know about them?" (how they feel.) She wanted Oliver to see it, and Miss Rogers led him down to the parlor, where they sat and talked some time about it. She said afterwards, "If I stopped my breath ten minutes I should die. What should you do if you should come to this room after I had been alone, and I had stopped my breath and died? Would you be sad? Would you like to have God stop your breath, and die to-day? When God wants you, how can he stop your breath?"

Dec. 21. Laura's fourteenth birthday; she asked me, "Do you like fourteen?" In writing an account of the story of yesterday, she had much difficulty, as she always does when she has to report a conversation between two or three persons; she becomes confused on the person and number of both pronouns and verbs.

Dec. 22. She finds more trouble with Section 15 than any she has had this term in arithmetic. She told me she dreamed that she went to Philadelphia with me to make a visit, and that she had a very good time. Her head was so full of it that she wanted to talk of my home, and to have me tell her " about all the furniture in it" and the rooms in each *story*, which word, thus applied, was new to-day. Next she wished to talk about going early to bed. She has been growing increasingly sensitive upon this point, and the birthday of yesterday has made her feel very much older. " I am large enough to sit up till eight." " Doctor thinks it is better for you to sleep much, and he knows best." " If Doctor knows best, why does not your (little) sister Lizzie go to bed at half past seven; your father (is a doctor) knows best? I think when I go to live with Doctor and Mrs. Howe in his house, I shall sit up till half past eight." She argued the point nearly an hour, and then was not convinced by my reasoning that she was not too old to go to bed at half past seven.

Dec. 23. She surprised me by doing eighteen sums When I told her how well she had done she made a very sad noise. I asked why. " I feel very sad that I did not do sums well yesterday and Thursday." She said this not because I had reproved her on either of these days, but because she is so ambitious that the distress at being obliged to delay on account of any new difficulty is great. She brought a feather of a peacock, and wanted me to tell her what a bird could do with such long feathers, the habits of the bird, and then we talked of parrots, and their speaking, which is a subject on which she is somewhat sensitive ; for it is a singular fact that while she expresses no feeling that men, women, and children can talk and she cannot, she always feels it when she learns of any of the lower animals speaking or hearing. Questioned her on the map that has North and South America upon it for the first time, asking miscellaneous questions, such as, " Which way is Cape Horn from Cape Farewell? " all which she answered without hesitation.

Visitors to the Institution will remember a very large globe, thirteen feet in circumference, which stands in the circular hall of entrance. Her success on the map made me desirous of testing her upon this.

I supposed that the convex surface would trouble her, and the raised lines were also different from those to which she was accustomed on the maps, but she was pleased when told she should have the rest of her lesson upon it. Her first remark was, " It is *too very* large." This expression was not a usual one, but neither qualifying word adequately expressed her idea of its size, so she used both. I placed her hand on the Russian

Possessions in North America, and moved it to Mexico, to give her an idea of the scale of distance. I then asked her to find the Gulf of Mexico, Hudson's Bay, etc., which she did at once, and indeed she found every place I called for, even to Boston. The blind children have never been able to do much on this globe in the first day's lesson, and I looked on with astonishment to see her fingers move so rapidly, scarce touching anything apparently but the spot called for.

When passing the globe recently the recollection of this lesson came freshly to my mind, and the wonderful feat, performed by touch alone, impressed me more than ever before.

Dec. 26. Another lesson on the globe; she found nearly all the capitals of the United States, and the chief cities of South America, and then of her own accord compared the Atlantic and Pacific to find their size, and asked to be taught the countries on the other side of the globe. This certainly shows very intelligent study of geography, but she had to be told it was best to learn first on the maps about the other continents, and then she could study again upon the globe.

Dec. 27. On Miss R.'s return after Christmas, Laura happened to be much interested in conversation with some one, and pushed her away when she attempted to speak to her. We thought it best to give her no opportunity to speak to her again for some time. To-day she asked, "Why does not Rogers come to see me?" I replied, "You can tell me why," and she at once confessed what she had done. After talking some time she said, "Why do you not send me to the House of Correction?" Last week I had read her a story about an idle boy who was sent there. She answered the question herself by saying, "You can send me to my chamber; that is my House of Correction." She said this very seriously, and was much troubled that she could not talk to Miss R.

Dec. 29. She has reached the tables of weights and measures in Colburn's Arithmetic, and learned Federal and English money. She commenced the map of Europe, taking Great Britain for a lesson.

Dec. 30. She talked about catamounts, panthers, and leopards, of which she had seen models yesterday. I asked her if she would like to live in the woods with them. "No, I should be sore because they would bite me so much. Would they eat me?" "If they were very hungry they would eat you for dinner." "Should I not go to heaven? I shall not see you in heaven. " "Why?" " I shall talk with my mouth." "Will you not talk with me?" "I shall be busy seeing strangers." It is not surprising that with the idea of her pleasure in heaven, should mingle that of being able to communicate with others than the little circle which surrounds her here.

CHAPTER XII.

January, 1844. Dr. Howe has been absent in Europe eight months to-day. Laura met me saying, "It is new happy year day." I wished her a Happy New Year, and she extended her hand to the east, spelling with her fingers the words, "Happy New Year," but added, with a laugh, "Doctor cannot know I say so."

Reviewed the tables which she learned last week, and added to them dry, ale, and wine measures Found it a very difficult matter to explain the difference between " want " and " wish " to her.

Jan. 2. Completed the tables this morning; when studying that of time, she asked, " How did men know that sixty seconds make one minute?" She had a call from a young lady who was deaf and dumb, but very graceful and pleasing in her manners. One would hardly suppose that Laura would perceive this with her one sense, but as soon as she had left she began to draw a comparison between Miss L. and herself, in which she acknowledged herself inferior. She perceived that some of the children were making New Year's presents yesterday, and desiring to imitate them she spent all her spare time in making " an apron for little Susan's doll, very nice and pretty, for a New Year's present."

Jan. 4. In her journal she wrote, " I thought about heaven and God, that he would invite me some time when he is ready for us to go to him. He made it storm very much." Advanced as far as Spain on the map of Europe, but she became so much interested in that country and its people that it occupied all the hour. She asked many questions about their dress. I told her of a Spanish girl I had seen at a concert, of her pretty dress and beautiful hair. " Did she talk English?" Told her I heard her say, " *Mui bien,*" to see if she remembered the words. I had told them to her long ago, as an example of Spanish, at the time she tried to read a Latin book. She said at once, " Very well," and then told me other words which I had said to her then. " Do they have the same animals in Spain that God made, that they do in England? Why do Spanish people come to America?"

Jan. 7. Laura's school had to be much interrupted to-day, on account of Miss J.'s illness. She bore this much better than she did when it occurred last week from my own illness, and was very sympathetic, anxious about her medicines, when they were to be taken, etc. To make me forget her unkindness at that time she has been very affectionate, telling me how much she loves me, and kissing and hugging me very often.

Jan. 12. She talked about dreams, and said, " Sometimes I dream about God." " What do you dream?" " I dreamed that I was in the entry, the round entry where Lurena was rolling in her chair (an invalid chair), and I went into a good place, that God knew I could not fall off the edge of the floor." This entry had an opening in the floor for the passage of light to the lower hall, around which was a railing, and I understood that in her dream she was within the rail, having tried to avoid the chair. Again she said, " I dreamed God took away my breath to heaven," accompanying the words with the sign of drawing something from her mouth.

In writing out a story which I had read to her, she remembered a sentence in it, which was, " You must thank the rabbit for your hat," meaning that it was made from the skin of a rabbit; but she took its literal sense, and stopped writing to say, " I cannot thank him; he cannot talk or know signs."

Jan. 13. She did but few sums, as she had forgotten about reducing fractions to their lowest terms. She wrote an account of the seal, and I found she understood it well, though read to her only once, and in almost the exact language of the encyclopædia. She is in a great hurry to get to Russia, probably because it is so extensive; she found the White Sea and rivers running into it without any help to-day.

Jan. 15. Laura did the sums which had puzzled her so much on Saturday as fast as I could myself. Her ability to overcome difficulties between two days is very peculiar, and she must think about them when she is sitting alone, for I never allude to arithmetic after the lesson is over, and she never asks me any questions, but it often happens that I leave her in a puzzle, and at the next lesson all goes smoothly.

Jan. 16. Yesterday Laura went to call on Miss Jeannette, who was visiting in Boston, and while I was absent spent her time in fault-finding. Eunice was wrong because she had girls come into her kitchen; Frank was wrong because he came over J.'s stairs to find Rogers. To each of these charges, which were evi dently made that J. might censure these persons, the answer was, she was very glad they came. " Swift is not nice, she put her dress on the bed," etc. About three months ago she did the same thing, and I talked with her a long time about it, until I thought she saw the wrong and felt sorry for it. When I called for her to take her home, she wanted to talk with me, but I told her 1 could not talk; that J. said she had been unkind, and I wanted her to think about it. She said no more, and soon after we got home it was time for her to go to bed. This morning at nine I told her I wanted to talk about it. She looked very sad when I asked her to tell *me* what she told J. In all the charges against Eunice and Frank, I showed her where they were both right in doing what they did : in reply to those she brought against myself, I told her of some careless things which she did yesterday when preparing to walk, such as pulling a dress down and leaving it on the floor, a closet door open, etc., and asked her if she would like to have me go to J. and tell of them that she might blame her ; and when I said that I shut the door, and hung up the dress, she answered, " You were kind, I was very unkind." I talked with her some time to convince her how often she might tell wrong stories, by blaming people for things she did not know about. She said, " Whose people did I blame? " I did not understand what she meant, and answered, "You blamed *many* people." " I blamed the Lord's people," said she. I was surprised at this, and asked, " What does *Lord's* mean ? " " God's, I saw it in a book," and she showed it to me in " The Child's Second Book," the Commandments, " I am the Lord thy God," etc. She said, " How can 1 ask

15

God to forgive me for blaming his people?" "You can ask him in your thoughts." "Can I know when he forgives me, how can I know?" "He will give you good thoughts." The next hour was for writing; she came to me and said, "I have asked God to forgive me, and I hope I shall not be unkind." She seated herself to write, but it was long before she could do so. I took a seat at a short distance from her and tried to read her conversation with herself, her soliloquy. She said to herself, "I am very sorry." "Doctor said he preferred to teach me himself." "Why cannot I know?" "It makes me very nervous." There was much more, but too rapid for me to read.

Jan. 17. Gave her a lesson in philosophy on the lever. She seemed to understand the three kinds, so that she could tell me what kind I used when taking coals with the tongs, ashes with the shovel, shutting a door, etc., and in one more lesson will do very well. After the lesson she said, "I think God has sent me good thoughts. I am very happy to-day; I do not feel cross any." I asked why she kissed me so much; she said, "Because I love you so much; you are very kind to teach me many new things."

Jan. 19. In the hour for conversation she introduced the subject of dreaming again. "Why does God give us dreams? Last night I dreamed I talked with my mouth. Did you hear me talk?" "No; I was asleep." "I talked as any people do in dreams." To the question, "What words did you dream?" I could get no answer. "Do Spanish people dream like us? Do they dream words like us?"

Jan. 20. We took a walk to Boston, and though

the thermometer was at 3°, and a high wind was blowing, Laura did not seem to mind it much. Reversed the usual order in geography by pointing her finger to the place, and asking for its name. A missionary from the West visited us, and said he had seen an Indian girl eighteen years of age, who was born deaf, dumb, and blind. She resides with her tribe in the northern part of Michigan State. Laura was much interested in her, and thought it would be a good arrangement for the girl to come here so that I could teach her. I suggested that she might teach her herself, and she was quite willing to do so. At the teatable to-night she amused herself by an imaginary conversation with Dr. Howe after his return. Holding out her hand to the chair at the table where he usually sat, she asked such questions as, '' Are you tired of going very far? Did you want to come back? '' At noon she asked Miss Rogers if Oliver knew about God. She looked very sad when Miss Rogers said no, and asked her why she did not teach him.

Jan. 24. When talking with J. she asked, '' When you ask God to give you good thoughts do you say, Lord, God, Father, My Heavenly, give me good thoughts? '' She probably got these words from some book. She asked also, '' When you look up do you see heaven? ''

Jan. 26. She was complaining much of the cold, and I took occasion to turn her thoughts to the poor, telling her of the sufferings of a family I had visited yesterday. Her first question was, '' Is God kind to the poor woman? ''

She completed the circuit of Europe, and now, to her

great delight, we have conversations on the objects of interest in the various countries, the people, their hab· its, articles of commerce, etc.

P. M. A large number of the representatives vis ited us. Laura had a very interesting conversation on their duties, asked them (through myself as interpreter) many very appropriate questions, and having fully under- stood the importance of laws, she asked if they sent them to Dr. Howe, that he might know what they were, and why they wanted the blind girls to go to the State House every winter.

Jan. 31. A very cold walk to-day. Laura com- plained but little, though she remarked, " It is like the northern parts of North America ; I think beavers could live here."

TWENTY-EIGHT OF JANUARY.

MY VERY DEAR DR. HOWE:

What can I first say to God when I am wrong? Would he send me good thoughts & forgive me when I am very sad for doing wrong? Why does he not love wrong people, if they love Him? Would he be very happy to have me think of Him & Heaven very often? Do you remember that you said I must think of God & Heaven? I want you to please to answer me to please me. I have learned about great many things to please you very much. Mrs. Harrington has got new little baby eight days last Saturday. God was very gener- ous & kind to give babies to many people. Miss Rog- ers' mother has got baby two months ago. I want to see you very much. I send much love to you. Is God ever ashamed? I think of God very often to love Him Why did you say that I must think of God? You must answer me all about it, if you do not I shall be sad. Shall we know what to ask God to do? When will He let us go to see him in Heaven? How did God tell people that he lived in Heaven? How could He take care of folks in Heaven? Why is He our Father? When can He let us go in Heaven? Why cannot He let wrong people to go to live with Him & be happy? Why should He not like to have us ask Him to send us good thoughts if we are not very sad for doing wrong?

Feb. 2. At nine, Laura asked, " Do you remember about the woollen gloves that I had two years ago, and that I hid them and told a lie about them, because I did not like them?" She talked of nothing but this the whole hour; said she was sorry she did so, and that the reason was, because she preferred to wear kid gloves. She spoke of her work yesterday, and I told her she was very industrious to knit so much. She appeared happy, and told me she would try to be very gentle all day, and not tire me, because I was weak and sick. At eleven we had an interesting lesson on the climates of Europe. At noon I was requested to take Laura to the school-room, as special company would be present. While waiting their arrival I was talking with her about the different kinds of coal, and the manner of making charcoal; we had just commenced the latter subject, when I noticed that she had left her handkerchief upon the desk. (At this time our dresses were not made with pockets, but as her handkerchief was in frequent use, she always carried it about with her.) She had been told repeatedly why it was not proper to leave it on the outside of the desk, and as she was so scrupulous in other matters of propriety, I supposed when she continued to do it, that it was from inadvertence, though I had noticed, within a few days, increasing impatience when reminded of it.   I paused in our conversation for an instant to say, "Put your handkerchief in your desk." She hesitated and put it in her lap, saying, "I prefer to put it in my lap," and held up her hand for me to go on with my story.   She knew that I objected to this because it was in the way when she had to leave her desk to go to the map.   I said, "I told you to put it in the desk, and now I want you to do it."   She sat still for about two minutes, and then lifted the lid very high, threw the handkerchief into the desk, and let it fall with such a noise as to startle all in the schoolroom.   Her face was growing pale, and she was evidently getting into a passion.   Whenever I have seen anything of this kind in the past year, the question, "Are you angry?" has always recalled her to her senses; but now she answered, "I am very cross"   I said to her, "I am very sorry, and I am very sorry you shut the desk so hard.   I want you to open it again, and take your handkerchief, and put it in gently." Putting on a very firm look, she said, "I will take it out to wipe my eyes, and put it back," meaning, "not to mind you."   I told her I wanted her first to put it in gently.   After a moment's hesitation, she took it out, let the cover slam as before, and then raised it to wipe her eyes.   I said, "No," decidedly, and gently took her hand down.   She sat still awhile, and then uttered the most frightful yell I ever heard.   Her face was pale, and she trembled from head to foot.   At this moment I heard the sound of visitors approaching, and only waited to say, "You must go and sit alone " A second she clung to my dress and then went quietly with me to her room.

At dinner-time I led her to the table, without speaking, and after that, gave her a chair to sit by herself, without work. Instead of looking troubled, as she generally does after having done anything wrong, she assumed an expression of indifference, talked to herself a little, and then feigned sleep. When she had taken tea, I asked her if she thought she could do what I told her to do this morning, if I let her go to the school-room. She said she would. I led her in and she did it very quietly. After this I talked an hour with her, trying to get her to feeling as she ought. She acknowledged the wrong at once, and said she was sorry, but her countenance indicated anything but sorrow. I left her during the hour for reading, and when I returned, she looked more troubled, and I told her she might go to bed, hoping that her own thoughts would bring her to a right state of feeling.

Saturday, Feb. 3. This morning have talked with Laura again, and am completely discouraged. I have tried every argument and appealed to every motive, with only partial success. The only thing which seemed to move her at all was, that I did not want to punish her, but that I could not let her do many things to-day to make her happy; when she went to exhibition I could not let Sophia talk with her, and could not let her go to the scholars' party in the evening, because only good girls went. But these were direct appeals to selfishness, and they were all that touched her. I did not know what to do, and never felt the need of counsel more. As I had exhausted every argument, I thought I would try the effect of a lesson in geography; so taught her something about the produce of different countries of Europe and of their manufactures. She was very quiet during this, and also a writing lesson which followed. The regular lesson for the last hour's school would have been the reading of a story, and I thought best to omit it. At dinner, she seemed to be very well satisfied with herself. When it was time to go into the school-room for the exhibition, she said, " I think I had better not go." I merely said, " It is time," and took her hand to lead her. During the exhbition she said, " Is Sophia here? " I told her she was in her desk in the school-room. " I am very happy," was the only reply. There was a spirit of defiance in Laura that I had never seen before. A few moments after, she attempted to kiss me, thinking she could take advantage of the presence of company. She answered questions readily and was willing to do what I wished her to do. At seven, I told her she could go to bed, and she went without any objection, but still with the same expression of countenance.

Sunday, Feb. 4. As Laura proposed that she should sit alone to-day, I left her this forenoon in the basement, where she had seated herself. When I returned from church, she did not appear to be troubled at all. I led her to dinner and then of her own accord she returned to the same place. At the tea-table she seemed much more sad, and after tea I sat down by her to try what effect I could produce then. I could now perceive a great difference, and after I told her how wrong it was that she did not feel more sad for doing wrong, she said, " I do feel very sad now. I was sad and cried this afternoon, and thought I was very wrong, and I asked God to forgive me and send me good thoughts and to love me." She then asked the old question, " What shall I ask God first, when I ask him to give me good thoughts? Must I say, ' Lord, Father, my Heavenly?' " I answered her that she could say just what she thought first. I told her that I was glad that she felt better now and that I would forgive her, and I hoped she would never be angry again. She said, " I think I *never* shall do so again. Why do I feel so very sad after I ask God to forgive me, and when you forgive me? " Told her because she felt so sorry she had done wrong at all.

If, in a faithful chronicle, the record of these last few days could have been omitted, it would be desirable both for Laura and myself. The remembrance of my anxiety to act wisely will never fade from my mind, but the experience of added years shows me that in those first few moments of excitement, it would have been wiser to have avoided the issue, and obtained submission in some other way. The fact that visitors were momentarily expected in the room, and the desire that no one should see Laura under such circumstances, added to the complications on my part.

I had felt for some time that a crisis was approaching, for, while there had been no act of positive disobedience, yet there was manifest to all who came in contact with her an inclination to submit to proper authority only after much argu-ment.

That a development like this should come as a parenthesis in a lesson in which she was much interested, and to which she was anxious to return, was a surprise, and the intensity of her feeling was not suspected by me, for I supposed I had only to say, " Are you angry ? " and that she would recover herself, as she had often done in previous times of excitement. Here was my error, and could I have seen the end from the beginning, I should not have asked the question, but have led her quietly to her own room, and left her to her meditations. The next step, unfortunately, devel-oped the worst features of the case, — a declara-tion of persistent disobedience, and the violent expression of passion, which was more like an ani-mal than a human being, followed by the assump-tion of an air of wilful indifference.

It will be seen that she rendered *literal* obedi-ence on the evening of the first day, but if I had accepted that, her own conscience would not have been satisfied, and although many may differ from me in opinion, I believe that all good effects of this trial on her future life would have been lost.

It was not a desire to obtain a passive obedience to my stronger will which led me to take the course I did at this time, but a thoughtful, unim-

passioned study of the case, and the conviction
that this was a crisis in which she was to conquer
herself, or ever after to be subject to her passions.
Painfully realizing my own inexperience and lack
of wisdom, with no one to share the responsibility,
the hours of waiting seemed days, and the days,
weeks. It would have been far easier to throw
my arms about her, and tell her how much sorrow
she was giving me, and then her sympathies would
have been touched, and, as had often happened
before, she would have yielded, only, however,
as before, to be overcome again very soon.

That she won the victory at last, and that hers
was a true repentance no one will doubt, and
when, with an expression which she could so well
give with her fingers, she said, "1 think I shall
never do so again," our tears flowed together, and
she did not doubt my love for her.

Monday, Feb. 5. Laura's arithmetic lesson was in
simple fellowship, and she performed the examples without difficulty. At nine gave her a lesson on the thermometer; explained the scale, mixed snow and salt to
show her how far the mercury would go down in the
tube She was delighted with the lesson, and led me
from room to room waiting in each to see its temperature. When she came for her writing lesson she asked,
" Why do I love you so very much to-day? "

Feb. 7. At this time Mr. Fisher was painting the
picture of Laura and Oliver, and while sitting with her
in his studio, I gave her a lesson on France. When

she found he had been there, she had many questions
to ask.

. *Feb. 8.* She was quite indignant when told in a lesson on bees that there were drones among them.

Feb. 12. In reading "The Harvey Boys," she found
the word "drunkards," and asked what it meant. A
long conversation followed on the effects of different
drinks, how men behaved who drank too much cider or
wine or rum or brandy. She said, "I want to talk a
long time about drunkards." Told her I did not like
to think or talk about them. "Will you talk about
crazy people? Will you talk about *dizzy* people?'
She has always confounded these two words, though
they have often been explained to her.

Feb. 13. Last evening Laura was in a very happy
mood, and before she went to bed she informed Miss J.
that she was going to *caper.* This word she had just
learned. Hearing a great noise, we went up quietly to
see what she was doing. We found her ready for bed,
but jumping from the bedstead and running to the next
room, then returning to do the same. This she continued half a dozen times and then threw herself down
exhausted. After resting, she commenced it again and
continued it for a quarter of an hour, occasionally stopping to see the effect on the sacking which held the bed,
and when she discovered that it was dropping down,
she laughed most heartily. Tired of this, she swung
her closet door violently on its hinges for five minutes,
until I feared she would suffer from cold, and spoke to
her to tell her it was time to go to sleep. It was a very
ludicrous scene, and I presume it was all suggested to
her by something which I had said when explaining the

word " caper." She had thought it over, and then decided she would try it herself. This morning I laughed with her about it and told her she must have a bed of iron if she wished to use it to jump upon, and that she must go up to bed at seven o'clock, so as not to disturb the girls who went to bed early. " I do not want to caper any more," she said. " I did it last night because I thought Doctor was coming so soon." I had told her that the young lambs capered to express their joy.

Feb. 23. She asked about jails, — if they had windows, etc., and then imagined herself there, and said, " What would you do if I had to go to jail? What would Doctor say?" etc. In her walk to the Point to-day, she was much interested in examining the blocks of ice which had been thrown one upon another by the tide. As it was low water, we could walk around among them. She showed that she had some appreciation of the descriptions of Swiss scenery that had been given her, by saying, " I think they are like mountains and glaciers."

Feb. 24. She is advancing very slowly now in arithmetic, her lessons being in the last miscellaneous examples in Colburn's Mental Arithmetic. Yesterday she succeeded in performing several and then found one which puzzled her, so it was left for this morning's lesson. This morning she had the answer ready for me, having thought it out by herself. She was much pleased with some of the visitors to-day, when told they were from Scotland, England, and the Azore Islands.

Feb. 26. For some time I have been desirous of knowing how much she remembered about words which

were taught her long ago, many of which she had probably never had occasion to use, and for a review decided
it would be a good exercise for her to take my old journal of two years ago. She liked the plan. We found
many words which she had forgotten, and some of which
she had very incorrect ideas, while there were many that
she explained perfectly, although she has never used
them.

Talking of families, she asked, "Are there families
in heaven?" I notice a marked difference in her manner of talking about the same words now; she asks so
many questions showing a great increase in intelligence.

Feb. 29. After working a long time she finished an
example in arithmetic, and when it was accomplished it
seemed so easy to her that she said, "I am very dull."
Having completed our "talks" upon the countries of
Europe, I gave her a review lesson on the boundaries
of all the countries, and was surprised to find what a
correct idea she had of their situation. She asked me to
define *pauper;* "the book says, there are nineteen hundred and sixty-nine paupers." The question "Where?"
showed that she had only read so much of the sentence,
but when referred to the book she replied, "In the
United States." It will be long, I fear, before she will
be able to read correctly, owing to this habit of taking
part of the author's meaning; but she enjoys reading
very much. She brought many words for explanation
from "The Harvey Boys." Vice was explained to her
as something wrong, and she said, "I viced last week."
As I was explaining the word "limbs" in its various
uses, she stopped me to ask, "How can God help hearing when I ask him to forgive me?" I had to tell her

that I did not want to talk about it until Dr. Howe answered her letters, and returned to the other subject, saying that the snow was falling fast, and the limbs of the trees were loaded with it. Another day, she as suddenly changed the conversation by asking, " How large is heaven? Is there a door to heaven? and how does the sky look? What is it made of?"

March 6 The deaf-mute pupils from the Hartford Asylum were to give an exhibition at the State House. Laura was told of it and that I was going to attend, and was very particular in her directions to me to see what *signs* they made, and to tell her. She has had a number of visitors who have been educated at Hartford, and is always much amused by the *signs* they made. As she has never been taught anything but the finger alphabet, of course their signs are without meaning to her.

March 7. We received notice that the Governor and Council, and Mr. Weld with his deaf-mute pupils, would visit us this afternoon, and as is always my custom, when there is to be any such unusual excitement for Laura, I prepared for this visit by taking a walk of five miles with her. I reported to her the exhibition yesterday, and told her how very well all the little girls behaved, and she said she should try to do as well to-day as the girls did yesterday. When they arrived, Laura had many questions to ask about Julia Brace, the deaf, dumb, and blind woman, who was here for a time, and in whom she was much interested. One of the girls asked her where she was brought up. As she did not understand that expression, she changed it to, " Where were you born?" Laura did not reply to her, but turned to me, and said quite indignantly, "I cannot remember when I was born." Mr. Weld, the teacher, talked to her some time, and as he was leaving her, said, "I love you and I will pray God to bless you." She immediately turned to me and said, "What is pray?" "To ask God." "What is bless?" "To give you good thoughts." Nothing more was said to me.

March 8. Laura appeared very thoughtful this morning, and said, when she came for her lesson, "Will it do any good for Mr. Weld to pray God to bless me?" She sat thinking for a while, and then said, "Will we be afraid to die?" I asked why we should be afraid to die. She replied, "Because we do not know any one," meaning in heaven. I saw she had not given me all her reasons, so repeated the question, and she said hesitatingly, "Because we cannot be very *sure* that God will want us. We cannot *know* that we have been *very* good when we live here, and we should be afraid he would not want us in heaven." I was surprised at this conversation, for she must have been thinking much upon the subject, and to be working out by herself many truths.

Governor Briggs asked her to write a letter to him. She was anxious that the writing should be very nice.

EIGHTH OF MARCH.

MY DEAR GOVERNOR:

I am very glad that you take care of people, & that you are very kind. Yesterday I sent Julia Brace a present to please her very much, & I hope that she will remember me for many years. She was here one year, & we all loved her very much. I was sad she went away & could never learn here any more. I should like to have you come to see me & the blind girls again when you can. Dear friend, good-bye.

March 11. She inquired into the cause of choking when drinking, and this opened the way for her first lesson in physiology. She had many questions to ask, as, "How can men know we have wind-pipes? Are they made of iron?" Asked her if she thought hers was iron, and she said, "No, flesh." Yesterday Miss Rogers came from church a few moments before 1 did, and found Laura reading "The Book of Psalms," and looking very pale and much excited. She said, "God is angry with the wicked every day. I was angry this year and last year, and I deceived Swift many times." Miss R. changed the subject, and got her interested in something else, but when I came home she began on the same subject: she said, "God will judge all people. What is judge?" I told her she could not understand all that book now, but that when Dr. Howe came home she would learn more. Her countenance brightened, and she said, "When are you going to teach me about God and heaven?"

March 12. Having walked to the city with Laura, found I could take her on board a brig just arrived from Lubec, Germany. While we were there the vessel moved from one part of the wharf to another. She expressed much fear that we should go too far, and asked me to "tell the men to throw the anchor." Had a very good opportunity to teach her many new words. The various parts of the ship, masts, ropes, cables, cabin, etc., as we were allowed to go about as we chose.

16

After getting home we talked it all over, so she might write an account of her visit to-morrow. Reviewed North America, which she remembers well.

March 13. Find she has forgotten more on South America than on any other map; but the wonder is she remembers as much as she does. In her lesson yesterday I told her we spoke of the sun as *he*, and to-day she asked, "Does *he* shine?" thinking that the improved way of asking the question. When telling me about some punishments that she received long ago, she said she was put in a closet, and asked, "Why do you not punish me so now? Why do my thoughts punish me now?" She is very industrious. and has knit four purses this week.

This is not a forced industry; indeed, it is hard to induce her to rest when we think she is weary. She takes up her work immediately on returning from a long walk, when most girls would think they had a good excuse for being idle, and even in the recesses, between the hours of school, she occupies every moment. At the beginning of the week she delights in making her plans, and wishes me to select the various colors of silk she is to use, so that she may lose no time in waiting for them. Once having told her how they are to be arranged I leave it entirely to her, and she rarely forgets, or has to ask me anything about them. If there is any new pattern or the style of work is to be changed, she learns it quickly, far more so than many do who can see, and she enjoys a variety.

March 18. At nine this morning she brought me a letter which she had written to Mrs. Morton, her old teacher. She has so much to say to her, and feels so sure that she will have no difficulty in understanding it. that she is very careless about the writing, and it took some time to correct all the mistakes. This I do, not upon the letters, but merely as a good exercise for her. When this was done, she produced a paper with the following words upon it : " perish, example, property, repeated, prince, lest, proverbs, afflicted, advice, recommend, poverty, wretched, chapters, pervert, an allusion, Jews, insensible, Romans, Saviour, offered, mingled, crucified, disgraceful, writer. Will you tell me what they mean?" she said. I told her I thought it would be best for her to ask me those that she could remember, rather than for me to read them from the paper to her, as she would remember them longer. Her custom is, after I give the definition, to frame a sentence and introduce the word. She began with " perish "; was told it meant to die, and said, " Betsy Smith perished last summer." Of " poverty " she said nothing in reply to the meaning given. " Romans " and " Jews " she understood easily about, but " advice " seemed to be harder for her. She asked, " Are ' advice ' and ' description' the same?" Left it for another time. " Offered, writer, disgraceful, and afflicted " she applied correctly at once. When told that I did not think she could understand Proverbs now, she said, " The Harvey boys said it "; and that she thought a reason that she should know it too.

I gave her the words " setting a good example and a bad example." She was much pleased with them, and said, " Frank set Susan* a very bad example yester-

---

* Two little deaf-mute children.

day; he opened the drawers and Susan rubbed his hand (a sign of wrong) and said he was wrong. That was a very bad example." This was one of the lessons that has no stopping-place, and she presses her questions upon me so rapidly that I am obliged to overstep the bounds of prudence, though I think it does her more injury to be held back than to gratify her desire for knowledge. When writing in her journal she told me she had used three new words, " neither, nor, and violently."

March 19. Reviewed yesterday's lesson, and found that many of the words she understood correctly, while of others, as " proverbs " and " advice," she got no correct idea. She asked the meaning of " prince," and wrote in her journal of the day, " God is a prince, because He takes care of his people." Commenced the maps of Asia, and she learned the boundaries of Sibe ria, the large rivers, rise and course, bays, seas, moun tains, and islands in the Arctic Ocean.

March 20. The whole hour was occupied in doing one sum, but as so often happens, she did all the diffi cult part very easily, and then got puzzled on a simple thing.

March 21. She did two examples, frequently com plimenting herself on her uncommon acuteness. One question was about the trees in an orchard: " One half the trees bear apples," etc.; she stopped to ask, " Did you ever eat any bear apples?" She had never hap pened to know any other use of that word but as the name of an animal, and probably supposed that the apples were a kind which bears liked to eat. Before he arithmetic lesson could go on it was necessary to explain, and give all the parts of the verb. Later in the day she talked of a lady whom she much admired, and thought she should like to be as graceful herself as Miss L., and tried experiments to see how well she could imitate her in bowing, courtesying, etc., but not very successfully.

March 22. Occasionally still there comes a feeling akin to jealousy, when she thinks of Dr. Howe's new relations; this morning she said, "Doctor loves his wife best of any." There was a cloud on her brow when she asked, "Does he love you like her?" which lifted considerably at my answer, though she said, "Why no, how do you know? I love him best of any, why does he not love me?" This feeling does not extend to Mrs. H. at all, for she always speaks of loving her very much, and is delighted with the letters she writes to her. The following is a copy of a letter written while she was anxiously waiting an answer to hers of January 28th.

24TH MARCH, 1844.

MY DEAR DR. HOWE:

I want to see you very much, I hope that you will come to South Boston in May. I have got a bad cough, for I got cold when I came home, in much snow with Miss Swift, but my cough is a little better. When you come home I shall be very happy to have you teach me in the Psalms Book,* about God and many new things I read in the Harvey Boys book, every Sunday. I am learning Asia now, I will tell you all about new things to please you very much. Why do you not write a

---

* The Book of Psalms was printed for the blind and bound in one olume.

letter to me often? Do you always pray to God to bless me? I think of you often. I send a great deal of love to you & Mrs. Howe. I shall be very happy to see you & her when you come home. I always miss you much. All the girls & I & Lurena had a very pleasant sleighing to a hotel. We had a nice drink of lemon & sugar & mince pie & sponge cake. Governor Briggs came twice to see us & the blind scholars. We are all well & happy & strong. I have not seen you for ten months, that is very long. I wrote a letter to Governor & he wrote a letter to me, long ago. Mr. Clifford is a doctor now to cure his wife. I wrote a letter to her. I want you to write a letter to me. Miss Swift sends her love to you. Are you in a hurry to see me & J. again? I would like to live with you & your wife in a new house, because I love you the best. All folks are very well and happy. I want you to answer my last letter to you about God & heaven, & souls & many questions.

My dear friend, good bye.

LAURA BRIDGMAN.

March 27. Completed Colburn's Mental Arithmetic.

At this time I did not realize what a remarkable work she had accomplished in a few days over a year, having commenced the book March 17, 1843. With the exception of two vacations of three weeks, and some few days of illness, she had had a daily lesson of three quarters of an hour. Having for many years since watched carefully the progress of other girls and boys of all grades of intellect, in the study of this same book, I should be inclined to-day to doubt my own journal, did I not find each day's work registered, so that with the book before me I can follow it step by step.

She was never allowed to leave any subject until she thoroughly understood it, and this was not accomplished by doing the work for her, but by putting questions to her which she could answer, and so gradually letting light in upon difficulties; she always went from her lesson feeling that she had performed the examples herself.

The effect of the mental discipline obtained from this study has been perceptible through all her life. Her feelings towards Mrs. Howe are shown in the following letter, dated —

APRIL 2, 1844.

MY DEAR MRS. HOWE:

I want to see you very much. I hope you are very well. I think of you very, very often. I was very much pleased to receive a letter from you and I liked it very much. When you come home, I shall shake your hands & hug & kiss you very hard, because I love you & am your dear friend. Are you very glad to receive letters from me? One night I dreamed that I was very glad to see you again. I hope you do not forget to talk with your fingers.

I am sad that people are very idle & dirty & poor (in Rome). My mother wrote a letter to Miss J. that she was very sick & my little sister was quite sick, but they are getting well. I am very well. I am your very dear friend. I try very hard about America & Europe & Asia & many other things. I learned philosophy long ago. I can say ship, paper, doctor, baby, tea, mother, father (mamma, papa), with my mouth. My teacher always reads a story to me; she is kind to me; she sets me a good example.

My dear friend, good bye.

April 3. When Laura came for her lesson she said, " My heart beats very quick, it is sick." " Long ago, when Miss Drew was my teacher, my heart beat quick and ached because I felt very sad that Adeline died, & I did not know about going to heaven." " Does that make your heart ache now?" " Monday I thought much about my dear best friend and *why* I should die; it made my heart beat quick, and I thought if I should know when He took my breath, & I tried to draw breath & could not. Do *you* lose your breath?" To change the conversation I replied, " Yes, when I run up stairs quickly." " I have lost part of the heart, it is not so large as it was when I was small." " Where did you lose it?" " I think it went to lungs. My blood ran quickly and made my heart beat very quickly."

April 8. Conversed with Laura about the railroad that is to be built from St. Petersburg to Moscow, telling her the Russians were going to have Americans to build it, the distance, expense, etc. She asked how the people could get four millions of dollars to pay for it. This introduced the Emperor Nicholas, his rank, office, and then she asked, " What is the man called who takes care of Americans?" Told her about the President, his name and residence, and asked her if she remembered Harrison. At the time of his death, seeing others with crape on their wrists, she made a band for herself. She remembered this, and asked why people wore it. This introduced the subject of wearing black in mourning, which she had never known anything about before. When speaking of Harrison I told her that people were sad because they could not have him to take care of them; she said quickly, "Were they sad that he went to heaven and was very happy there?" In geography her lesson was on China, and she was delighted to hear of the strange customs of the people, expressing much surprise, especially at their manner of reading from right to left, the great wall, etc.

April 11. Gave her a lesson on the discovery of America by Columbus, the part of the continent which he found, and commenced the account of the colonies; but history has so many dark pages that I find it difficult to tell her a connected story without alluding to wars, and this would be so terrible to her that I cannot think of beginning it at present.

April 18. She reviewed three sections in arithmetic very successfully. She has been reviewing the last miscellaneous examples, and had to study on some of them some time before getting them right, having forgotten her former work, but this was not more noticeable than with all the other girls. For a review of Europe and Asia took her to the great globe, and as before, she found all the localities readily.

April 19. She was in an ecstasy of delight, hugging me almost to suffocation because she was to begin the map of Africa. What the special attraction of this map is, I cannot find, but she has been looking forward to it with great anticipations.

CHAPTER XIII.

LAURA received to-day Dr. Howe's reply to her letter of January 28.

MY DEAR LITTLE LAURA:

Mrs. Howe has a sweet little baby; — it is a little girl; we shall call her Julia; she is very smooth and soft and nice; she does not cry much, and we love her very, very much. You love her too, I think, do you not? But you never felt of her, and she never kissed you, and how can you love her? It is not your hands, nor your body, nor your head, which loves her and loves me, but your soul. If your hand were to be cut off, you would love me the same; so it is not the body which loves. Nobody knows what the soul is, but we know it is not the body, and cannot be hurt like the body; and when the body dies the soul cannot die. You ask me in your letter a great many things about the soul and about God; but, my dear little girl, it would take very much time and very many sheets of paper to tell you all I think about it, and I am very busy with taking care of my dear wife; but I shall try to tell you a little, and you must wait until I come home, in June, we will talk very much about all these things. You have been angry a few times, and you have known others to be angry, and you know what I mean by anger; you love me and many friends, and you know what I mean by love. When I say there is a spirit of love in the world, I mean that good people love each other; but you cannot feel the spirit of love with your fingers; it has no shape, no body; it is not in one place more than in another, yet wherever there are good people there is a spirit of love. God is a spirit, the spirit of love. If you go into a house, and the children tell you that their father whips them, and will not feed them; if the house is cold and dirty, and everybody is sad and frightened, because the father is bad and angry and cruel, you will know that the father has no spirit of love. You never felt of him, you never had him strike you, you do not know what man he is, and yet you know he has not the spirit of love; that is, he is not a good, kind father. If you go into another house, and the children are all warm, and well fed, and well taught, and are very happy, and everybody tells you that the father did all this, and made them happy, then you know he has the spirit of love; you never saw him, and yet you know certainly that he is good, and you may say that the spirit of love reigns in that house. Now, my dear child, I go all about in this great world, and I see it filled with beautiful things, and there are a great many millions of people, and there is food for them, and fire for them, and clothes for them, and they can be happy if they have the mind to be, and if they will love each other. All this world, and all these peo-ple, and all the animals, and all things, were made by God. He is not a man, nor like a man; I cannot see him, nor feel him, any more than you saw and felt the good father of that family; but I know that he has the spirit of love, because he too provided everything to make all the people happy. God wants everybody to be happy all the time, every day, Sundays and all, and to love one another ; and if they love one another they will be happy ; and when their bodies die, their souls will live on, and be happy, and then they will know more about God.

The good father of the family I spoke to you about let his children do as they wished to do, because he loved to have them free ; but he let them know that he wished them to love each other and to do good ; and if they obeyed his will they were happy ; but if they did not love each other, or if they did any wrong, they were unhappy ; and if one child did wrong it made the others unhappy too. So in the great world. God left men and women and children to do as they wished, and let them know if they love one another and do good they will be happy ; but if they do wrong, they will be unhappy, and make others unhappy likewise.

I will try to tell you why people have pain sometimes, and are sick, and die ; but I cannot take so much time and paper now. But you must be sure that God loves you, and loves everybody, and wants you and every-body to be happy ; and if you love everybody, and do them all the good you can, and try to make them happy, you will be very happy yourself, and will be much hap-pier after your body dies than you are now.

Dear little Laura, I love you very much. I want you to be happy and good. I want you to know many things, but you must be patient and learn easy things first and hard ones afterwards. When you were a little baby, you could not walk, and you learned first to creep on your hands and knees, and then to walk a little, and by and by you grew strong, and walked much. It would be wrong for a little child to want to walk very far before it was strong. Your mind is young and weak, and cannot understand hard things, but by and by it will be stronger, and you will be able to understand hard things, and I and my wife will help Miss Swift to show you all about things that now you do not know. Be patient, then, dear Laura; be obedient to your teacher, and to those older than you; love everybody and do not be afraid.

Good by! I shall come soon, and we will talk and be happy. Your true friend,

DOCTOR.

This letter was read twice to her, but she made no conversation upon it, nor did she ever allude to it afterwards. Although she understood each separate word, I think the argument was beyond her capacity. She was much excited on hearing of the baby, and pleased with her name.

In four lessons she completed the tour of Africa. For some time she has yielded to her inclination to utter disagreeable sounds more frequently than before, and I tried to have her understand the bad effects of such noises on others. She argued in their favor, saying, "I have very much voice, God gave me much voice." We compromised the matter in this way: she is to make no noises until half past one, and then, for an hour, she is to shut herself in her room, and make as many as she wishes to.

April 29. Yesterday, Laura occupied herself in writing letters, and I noticed that she had dated them all wrong. She insisted upon its being the thirtieth to-day, " because April has thirty days, and Doctor went a year ago the first day of May and that was Monday, so Sunday was the last day of April." Her process of reasoning was very amusing, and would have been all right if this year had not been Leap Year, which she had never heard of before. One of our visitors wished me to tell Laura that he was from Wales. She was very ready in answering his questions, and telling him what she knew about his country.

May 30. Many of the scholars were to go to Boston to enjoy the sounds of the great temperance procession, and I thought it a good time to give Laura a lesson on that subject. She has been much interested in it since she read " The Harvey Boys," and found there was such a thing as a drunkard. When I told her how many men would walk, she remembered the celebration of the 17th of June, and said, " I can go and feel the drums." She asked if they had anything beside drums, and made a sign of drawing the bow, not knowing the word violin, and told me she thought the bow was made of the tail of some animal. " Why do the people walk?" Told her it was to show that they did not drink rum or brandy. " That is right, we cannot have any men that love to drink such liquors." It was. a mystery to her how so many men happened to come to Boston at once. Explained to her that the friends of temperance in Boston invited those from other towns to come, and have a great meeting, and that Gov. Briggs would ride in a carriage with four white horses. She was sure she never knew there were white horses, and asked if they would not get soiled quickly, lying on the ground. One of her questions was, " Do poor people walk in the procession? How can they walk without any shoes?" Some time ago I had told her about a poor family, and that the children had no shoes, therefore she thinks that all poor people have no shoes. When talking about the Pyramids, I said they were made 2800 years ago. " They are in heaven now," she said. Supposing she referred to the Pyramids, I asked, " What are pyramids?" " Houses made of stone. I mean the men who made them are in heaven."

June 3. According to a promise made last week, I took Laura into the music-room to let her examine the various instruments. When shown the orphy-clyde, she said she thought the mouth of it would be a good bath-tub for baby Julia. Whenever she struck the drums or triangles, she varied the time in her beats, and her perception of this, through the effect of the vibrations upon her sense of feeling, is evidently what gives her pleasure. She showed much enjoyment when the procession was passing, and talked as if she could hear the music. She was talking with Miss Jeannette about impatience, and said, " I am impatient with you and with my teacher, but I am never impatient with Doctor." " Why not?" she asked. " Because I never like to let men see me impatient."

June 7. She asked me, " Why does it not rain in Egypt?" I told her I thought she could not understand about that now, and she said with a great deal of feeling, " I am too old for you to tell me I cannot under stand. I can understand hard things now."

June 10. At nine she was full of a project for her doll, and in a great frolic over it. Little Frank has a doll dressed as a boy, and Laura named him Mr. Deter; she says he is going to marry her doll. She told of the plan this morning, and was in a great hurry to wash her closet, which she calls " Jenner's house," so as to have everything in order before Wednesday. "It is so very nice to get all things ready. Do you not think the doll will be much happier, because Dr. Howe said he was much happier to be married?" I laughed, but she did not like it. She gave me an invitation to be present at the wedding. I asked who would marry them, and this gave her a new idea, as she did not know it was customary to have a minister. Finding she did not know all about it, she said. "I wish you would be married, and then I would see you, and know what the minister said." I told her she must ask Jenner if she would love and obey Mr. Deter, if she wanted to say what the minister did. She laughed heartily at this and said, "I think she will, for she is always kind and obedient." She could hardly wait for recess to come to commence her preparations, and all day has talked to every one she met about it. For a long time she had not cared at all for her doll, but now thinks of nothing else.

June 11. Her writing is a source of much trouble, for all her practising on separate letters seems to avail so little; as soon as she begins to write sentences, she returns to the same bad style. Not so her geography. As she had completed all the maps, I led her to the globe, put her hand on Lake Superior, and asked her to find Cairo. She thought an instant, and said, "Africa is southeast from North America," and her finger was on the little pin denoting it. She answered every question all over the world with perfect ease, while I looked on with wonder. She was imagining herself in my position to-day, and said, "If I was teacher and you were a little girl and you got angry, I should put you in the closet, and I should be sad and have you sit alone."

June 17. Finding my head bandaged when she came for her lesson, she said, looking much troubled, "Your head is so very hot I know you will have a fever"; and she wanted me to promise her that I would ask Dr. Fisher to let her come into the room if I was sick. "I will be your nurse and take care of you, and in the night sometimes I will sit up with you. Are you willing?" This plan was so novel that she was delighted with the prospect. In the recess, when she was alone by herself, a company of soldiers passed, and when she came for her lesson she asked what it was, for she had *felt* them. We talked about military uniforms, colors, etc.

June 19. We walked to the green-house at the Point. This is the first season she has ever perceived the smell of a rose or pink, and now she puts all flowers to her nose, and is disappointed if they have no perfume. The gardener gave her many flowers, and among them some lemon verbena; she smelled it and pushed it from her, saying, "It smells like varnish." Explained the word "guilty" to her and she asked, "Did you not see many little boys that looked *guilty* when you went to the Correction House that you told me about long ago?"

June 25. She completed to-day a letter to Mrs. Howe in reply to one she had just received, describing

17

her visit to Vesuvius. It is quite in advance of any she has previously written, so I give it entire.

MY DEAR MRS. HOWE:

I was very much delighted to receive a very long letter from you. I understood about lava & crater. I was much surprised to hear about new things. I do not know how to knit a pair of shoes for your dear little Julia. I love your baby very much, & am your precious. (She is my precious.) I shall make a present for you to remember me many years. I should like to live with you and your husband & dear baby. While you were away one year I was in great misery, & had to miss you many times. I did not like to have you go away with Dr. Howe. As soon as you come home, I shall run to you & kiss & hug you very hard, & shall take my very dear baby & kiss it very softly & take off her things. I shall always set her a good example. I want to see her very much. I should like to make a very nice clothes to help you. I know Vesuvius very well, for Miss Swift taught me about it a long time ago. I can smell roses much better than I did two years ago, & it gives me much pleasure in smelling roses. I like them very much. I am very happy that you are coming very soon to see me. I shall walk with you & talk about many things. Miss Jenner was married to Mr. Deter (two dolls) two weeks ago, on Thursday evening. I was a minister to marry them. My friends went to a wedding. Mrs. Deter had wedding cake for them after she was married. Mrs. Deter loves her husband very much & best, & is very happy with him. Did you like to ride on mule's back

np the mountains? Were you afraid of them? You
will please to write a letter to me some time if you can.
Miss J. is very well & happy. I am happy that Julia
is so happy to see the bright light. I want you to come
back *now;* if you do not come quick, then I must send
a long string to pull you over the sea to South Boston.
I thought of you & Julia & Doctor many times, that
they would love me very much, because I love them
& you so much. I always go to Boston with my
teacher for exercise. It makes my health more better
& strong Did mule have saddle on his back? Tell
Doctor that I cannot write another letter to him because
I have much to write to you, so I have not time to write
to him, but he can see what your letter says. Give my
love to him. I send a great deal of love to you & a kiss
for baby. On the fourth day of July we are going to
have dinner in the school-room. I am very sad not to
have you come & have a very nice dinner with me &
have some many pretty flowers. I wish you could come
very much. Please to kiss the baby for me many times
a day, every day. My best friend, good-bye.

June 28. Laura said this morning, " How many
countries must send us things to make all the things in
this house?" She talked an hour, answering such questions as, What do the Southern States send us? What
the Western, South America, Russia, France, England,
China? etc. She is very quick in her replies

July 1. Laura examined an æolian harp which I
had had given me, and asked me to play upon it.
When told that the wind played upon it she was impatient to have it play that she might *feel it.* I put it in

the window and placed her hand on the wooden side, but told her I thought there was nothing which she could feel. She sat very still for several minutes; when a puff of wind gave the first note, she started, and said, "It is like the organ." It happened to be a low note, and was so much like the organ that I thought some one must be playing in the room below. Next, the wind struck a high note, and she said, "That is like singing." I tried to feel it, but told her I could only feel a *very, very* little. She said, "Is it like very small animals that you can only see with a spy-glass?"

July 8. Commenced a story called "Life in the Desert." It is much longer than those I have read to her, and will take six readings to complete it. The style is very different also, but I selected it on account of her great interest in Africa. When I read to her about the tribe of Tuaricks killing the Tibboos, she was horror-struck, and did not seem to know what to say about it. It was the first time she had ever heard of one man killing another.

A cotton-pod half opened, showing the cotton on the seeds just ready to be gathered, led me to tell her something about the slaves in the Southern States. She asked if they were Tibboo people that were brought from Africa, but said nothing about the wrong of keeping them as slaves, which I thought might occur to her.

Aug. 6. Laura was puzzled to find the interest for a certain number of days, and assured me the only reason she could not get it right was because there were Latin words in the question, "per cent." She has understood this a long time. She is getting almost work-crazy, she is so anxious to complete a certain number of purses each week. She tells me each day how much she can do, and is displeased if interrupted.

Aug. 19. In our hour for conversation, she asked if she ever told me about her friends at home, and gave me an account of the time she lived at home. It consisted chiefly of a description of all the animals on the farm. One was three feet high and covered with hair, curled like a sheep. She was sure it could not be a sheep. She said she was very much frightened when her mother opened the cover of a hair trunk as she thought it was an animal. I asked her what she used to think about when she lived at home. She said, " I could not think or talk good then. I did not know any of my friends in Pearl Street,* Boston then." I asked her if she thought how kind her mother was. She said, " No, I did not think she was kind, for she whipped me and shook me." Explained to her why she had to do it, and the trouble she caused her mother, and in reply she told me how she used to pinch her mother when she wanted anything.

Aug. 24. I told her she might write a story herself, just as gentlemen and ladies wrote in the books which I had read to her. She was delighted and said she would try, but I must not look at it until it was finished. At the close of the hour she brought me the following, being her first attempt : —

" There was a little girl named Jane Damon, who lived in the country with Mrs. Damon. She was very good & amiable, & was never cross any. Jane Damon always obeyed her mother. One day she went

---

* At the time she came to the Institution it was in Pearl Street.

with her mother to see her friends, and they went to see beautiful flowers in the garden. When Mrs. Damon told Jane, you must go to school, she got ready as fast as she could. She had the books & writing in her own desk. Her teacher was very kind to her scholars. Her name was Miss Charlotte. Mrs. Damon gave Jane a beautiful present. Her sister asked what it was, & her mother said it was a ring called diamond stone. After a few days her mother took Jane to see her grandmother, and staid for one week. She had a very pleasant visit. Mrs. Damon had a little girl named Clara Damon, & Jane took good care of Clara while her mother was away a little while. She did not cry any for some milk, but Jane fed Clara with a spoon; she loved her so very much."

Aug. 26. Speaking of her health, she said, "I was sick last year, and my mind was dizzy, and I was much frightened in my head." She asked the meaning of " insensible " and " crucified." The latter I defined as meaning to make a cross. Her application was, "Jane Damon crucifies the wires of her basket and winds the worsted on them." I was obliged to tell her that she did not quite understand it, and had better not use it. The next word was " mingle," which I defined " mix," but found she did not know that word either. When explained, she said, " The drunkard mixes sugar and rum to drink." The next was " mock." From these words I knew she had been reading about the crucifixion, but had failed to get any idea of it on account of so many of the words used being unintelligible to her. She wished to prove to me she did not forget words, and said, " Perish is to die, you told me last winter, and machine — my writing-board is a machine to write with; require, is when I tell you, you must mend my stockings; I require you to do them. I require you to read my story to Jane Damon."

In geography she is studying the zones on the globe.

Sept. 3. Completed the review of the last half of Colburn's Arithmetic, and now is to take up written arithmetic. She was very happy in welcoming Dr. Howe on his return from Europe, but was not so much excited as she would have been if Mrs. Howe and the baby had accompanied him from New York.

Sept. 5. Lesson on latitude, calculating it in miles as well as degrees. She said, " My mother lives one hundred and twenty miles north of us, that is two degrees," and added, " Hanover is by the Connecticut River: why do I not go in a boat?" Asked her to tell me how she could go. Her first thought was, that she could get to the Merrimac, and in some way across to the Connecticut. When told there was a way to go by water, but she must get into the boat in Boston Harbor, after much thinking, she said, " I must go by Cape Cod and then sail through Long Island Sound to the Connecticut River."

Sept. 12. The baby, which had just arrived with its mother, Mrs. Howe, was her only thought. She took no interest in her lessons, but could talk of nothing but what she planned to do for little Julia, the first thing being to give her all her playthings.

.

CHAPTER XIV.

Nov. 1, 1844. A vacation of three weeks has just passed, and Laura has much to tell of what she has seen, " so many new things." Among these were a woollen factory and a grist-mill, and of both she gave me very good descriptions. I was surprised to find how much she had understood and remembered. When she did not know the name of any part of the work, she made signs imitating the people at work, so that I could guess what it was. She asked why the meal was so hot after it was ground, and we had a talk about friction, which I illustrated, much to her satisfaction, by rubbing two pieces of wood together. Her greatest exploit, however, was that she had ridden on a donkey, and this she told of with great glee.

Nov. 15. Dr. Howe gave her a lesson last evening on the use of " ful " and " less." He thought she understood it perfectly, but her report of it to-day is a good illustration of the difficulties we meet with. She said, " Doctor talked to me about ful and less. I am motherful and sisterful ; you are brotherless. Rained is a derivative word ; rain is a primitive. Is it derivative to-day?" Told her I did not know what she meant. She explained it, " Is it rainy to-day?"

I taught her the force of the prefixes " un " and " in " and the new words " need " and " harm."

Nov. 18. She came this morning for a lesson, bringing a list of words written on a paper which she had found in a book yesterday. Explained " security, crime, commit, thus, propriety, constantly, character." She wished to have " profane " explained ; I told her profane talking was when any one used bad words. She thought a moment, and said, " Mr. T." (an old man) " talks profane words, because his head is bad, and he cannot know." Told her he talked silly words, but that " profane " was not a good word for her to use. because she did not understand it; it did not seem best that she should be told at present of any more of the sins of man. Later in the day explained " fully, satisfied, chance, opportunity, and immediately," and then talked with her about my plan of going home to live in the spring. She said, " I shall get a string and tie your hands to prevent you from packing your trunk." She expressed her sorrow that 1 must ever go away, and said, " I must be with you all the time now ; I hope when you are in heaven you will be very glad to see me. If we are very sick we must be patient, and ask God to invite us. Dr. Howe told me that Orrin was so very gentle God wanted him earlier, and Adeline too."

Nov. 20. Spent an hour in reviewing the fifty new words she has learned in a week, and found she remembered nearly all, and introduced them into sentences very correctly. In defining " sunbeam " she said, " When I stand by the window and feel the end of the sun it is a sunbeam."

Nov. 25. Another long list of words, " pretend, confess, conceal, conduct, diligent." Of these " pre-

tend " was the most difficult. They occupied an hour,
and for another lesson, " appear, confidence, offending,
and encourage."

Dec. 2. Laura said, " ' The Child's Book ' says we
must turn our knowledge to some profit: what does
that mean?" There was so much in this idea that it
took a long conversation to explain it. " Possess "
was defined as " to have." Example, that she possessed some knowledge now, and I hoped she would
possess much more at the end of a year. She said,
" Yes, I hope I shall of English Reader and Psalms,
and the Bible."

Dec. 9. She asked, " Do crazy people talk profanely
when they dream, but not think?" Three weeks since
I had told her she would never have to use this word,
but she is determined to find what it means if possible,
and so whenever she meets with a word she thinks is
not good, she asks if it is profane. New words to-day
were " suspicious, suspect, anticipate, hateful." She
counted the months that I should teach her, and
talked of her new teacher. " I hope you will teach her
how to talk with her fingers, and what things to teach
me, and I hope Doctor will tell her what she must teach
me. She must not talk about heaven to me, because
he says I must wait for him to tell me about that."

In the geography lesson we had a long talk on the
subject of the Chinese ports being shut to foreigners.
She could not see why the Chinese should be suspicious
of Americans, though she thought they might be of the
Tartars or Siberians, but not of us. She was much
surprised to hear of the size of their cities, and asked.
" How *very* long will it take to count them?"

Dec. 12. Laura is enjoying imaginary shopping, with a purse full of silver to pay for it, as an exercise in arithmetic. She says, "It is much nicer than the book was."

She asked, "What do bescond and Matthew chap. mean?" Taught her "abscond," and about "chapters" and "verses," also "possibly, prophets, text, occasion, stumbling." She said, "The drunkard's brains are dizzy so that he stumbles." This subject, though repulsive to her, seems to fascinate her so she is constantly drawing her examples from it.

Dec. 19. As she is very prompt in settling her bills in dollars and cents, I had her try to reckon in shillings and pence. She is familiar with fractions, and so will probably find little difficulty. She read the word "abound" in her lesson, and I asked if she knew it. "Yes, my head abounded when it struck the wall in my mother's house."

We had a long discussion on the word "always," which she was so sure she understood correctly that she was at first unwilling to accept my criticism on her use of it. She insisted that she was "always in the parlor" and "always in her closet," meaning at some time *every day* she was there. Probably when I first gave her the word I defined it *every day.*

Jan. 21, 1845. Laura knit a very pretty purse and sent to the Mechanics' Fair. The committee awarded her a diploma and medal. I read it through to her and she seemed frightened at the number of unknown words, but was much pleased when she had learned them all.

Jan. 22. Dr. Howe had been giving Laura some

lessons in grammar on nouns and adjectives, and I took up the subject for regular lessons to-day. She had already learned nouns and adjectives so she rarely made a mistake on them. I took up pronouns, and told her "you" and "me" were pronouns, and I wanted she should think of other words we used to mean herself and myself, and she gave me very quickly all the cases of the pronouns "I" and "you." I then gave her an example in which *it* occurred, and she named it as a pronoun. In the sentence, "The plants look very pretty, and they must have much water to make them grow," she told correctly the part of speech of all the words but three, — the, very, and to. Gave her the sentence, "The sun is not shining," to teach her articles and participles. In the sentence, "It is not good weather," she said, "I do not know *it*, I think it does not stand for a noun." Another sentence was, "I hope you will be able to go to the city to-day." She gave all the words correctly until she came to to-day, and first called it an adjective and then a noun, but was not satisfied with either.

Feb. 3. She finds quickly every place that is put down on the raised map of Europe, cities, towns, rivers, mountains, etc. In grammar she learned the kinds of nouns and gender, having learned number in a previous lesson.

Feb. 10. In parsing a sentence she gives the kind of noun, its person, number, and gender, also of pronouns. The new words to-day were "elegant, apparel, exhibit, plan. conveyance, cheerful. elevating, avoid, frivolous, gloomy, desirable, style." After I had explained the last two she said, "It is desirable for us to live in style"

I asked her what style she thought most desirable. Her answer was that " It makes us happier than to be killed," showing she appreciated the first words of the sentence, but did not connect the last two understandingly.

Feb. 13. After a recess she came to me with her apron unfastened, and said, turning to me to hook it, " Do something to deserve to be thanked." I had lately taught her the word " deserve." Gave her a review lesson upon nouns. She was very quick in her answers, and wished me to be faster in telling her new things, " Because if you do not, you will not have time to teach me all about grammar before you go away, and a new teacher will not know how to teach grammar."

Feb. 18. Gave Laura a ciphering-board, and had her commence with numeration. It is two years since she has done anything with the board, and she has forgotten a good deal. She was troubled on account of a new arrangement, by which part of my time is to be devoted to teaching Oliver. It is not strange that she should dislike it, she has so long had undivided attention, and she finds her plans for accomplishing a certain amount in her studies will be interfered with. This was made necessary by the resignation of Miss Rogers, who has been his teacher.

March 5. Oliver wished to remain with me while I gave Laura a lesson. As soon as she perceived he was in the room, she wanted to talk with him. She has adopted lately a peculiar style of conversation. She tells him a number of stories, all imaginary, but upon subjects that she knows interest him, and when he appears to be sufficiently troubled, she tells him, " I am in fun, I say it for fun." Although she has done it repeatedly he is deceived each time, but takes it in good part, and is still willing to talk with her.

March 12. One of our visitors was going to the Cape of Good Hope soon, and Laura sustained her part in a conversation with him very creditably, asking the length of voyage, about the climate, productions, etc.

March 24. The new words for to-day were "ingratitude, feeble, control, controllable, accomplish, instruct, instructor, instructress." The effect of learning so many new words is quite noticeable in her language. She is very ambitious to use as many of them as possible, and throws aside those which we are in the habit of using in ordinary conversation to substitute others which she finds in books. The consequence is that her language to-day is more faulty than it was six months ago, and is best described as language *on stilts.* Greater familiarity with books and careful attention to her conversation will do much to correct it, but I fear it will always have many peculiarities.

Dr. Howe remarks on this subject in his Thirteenth Report : —

"In truth, people seldom stop to reflect upon the nature of arbitrary language, upon its essential importance to the development of the intellect, or upon the wonderful process by which we gradually advance from the power of naming single objects to that of condensing many of them into one complex term, — from the alpha of language, mamma, up to its omega, universe !

"How much is asserted in the simplest sentence, as this, for instance : ' We might have been more truly

happy had our widowed father remained contentedly
with us.' Here is the assertion of the plurality of
persons ; of their condition in past time ; of the fact
of their having been moderately happy in the society of
their father ; there is the negation of their entire happiness ; the implied doubt whether after all they would
have been happier ; their relation as children ; their regret
at their father's departure. Of the other person it is
directly affirmed that he had been with his children ; it
is implied that he had been married ; that he had lost his
wife, not by separation, but by death ; that he was not
contented to remain with his children ; that he had gone
away from them ; that he might have remained with
them, etc., etc.

" When we reflect upon that principle of the mind
which requires that all possible objects, qualities, and
conditions must be linked so closely with signs that the
perception of the signs shall recall them necessarily and
instantly ; and when we consider how much is attained
by young persons, who a few years ago could hardly
master baby's prattle, but who now have all the vast
sweep of thought, the great amount of knowledge, the
degree of reflection, of separation, and of generalization
necessary to comprehend such a phrase as,

'Count all the advantage prosperous vice attains,
'T is but what virtue flies from, and disdains,'

we may say with the ancient, ' There is but one object
greater than the human soul, and that one is its
Creator.'

" The space between the starting-point of the infant
and that obtained by the mature man is immense ; but

our minds. aided by language which gives to them wings, skim swiftly and delightedly over the whole, as the wild fowl flies from zone to zone ; while Laura is like one of those birds shorn of its wings, and doomed to attempt the vast distance on its weary feet. If persons will only make these reflections they will be inclined rather to wonder that she has gone so far than to feel surprised at her not having gone farther."

March 30.   She repeated to me this morning the story of the birth of Christ, and of his being carried away because of a bad governor, which Dr. Howe had told her yesterday.

April 22.   In arithmetic she has advanced to reduction.   One question was about duties in a custom-house, a subject which was all new to her, and we spent an hour in the explanation of freight, imports, exports, etc.

When shown a calla lily, she compared it to a horse's ear, and said the stamens had a very fine nap on them. Counting the days before I was to leave her, she said, "Your time runs so very fast, like a balloon."

April 30.   Completed Abbott's story of " Marco Paul in Boston," which we have been reading at intervals for several months, much to her enjoyment, also finished the seventh section of Colburn's Sequel.

Dr. Howe gives in his Thirteenth Annual Report some extracts from his own journal, showing his method of conversing with her on religious subjects.

" In talking with Laura to-day on the subject of the Deity, I said, ' How do men make bread?' ' From wheat.' 'How do they make wheat?' 'They can-not make wheat,' said she. 'Then how do they get it?' said I. 'God makes it grow.' 'Why?' 'For man to eat,' said she. I then explained to her that some birds and animals eat grain, and asked, 'Why does God give it to them?' She said, 'To make them happy.' 'But does he love them?' said I. 'No,' said she, 'they have no souls.'

" I then told her there are some beautiful islands on the globe, where the sun shines clearly and warmly; where there are rich meadows and sweet flowers and tall trees and shady groves; where the brooks run merrily down the hills, and where there is plenty of delicious fruit and nutritive plants; that these islands are never visited by man, yet nevertheless that thousands of birds are singing in the branches, and rejoicing over their little ones; that the young animals are frolicking on the soft grass, and the old ones looking on them with silent joy; that the fishes are swimming briskly about in the clear streams, and leaping out sportively into the air, and that all this has been going on thousands of years.

" After thus trying to give her as vivid a picture as I could of the happy inhabitants of these peaceful isles, I asked her who made such beautiful places. She said, 'God' 'But for what did he make them?' 'To make the animals all happy,' said she, and added of her own accord, 'God is very good to make them hap-py.' She then meditated a little, and said, 'Can they thank him?' 'Not in words,' said I. I then went on to show her that he had no need of thanks in words; that he did not do these good things in order to be

18

thanked, when she stopped me by asking, 'Why he did not give them souls?' I tried to explain how much of reason and sense they really possess, and how grateful all of God's children should be for what they have without asking why it was not more, when she said suddenly, 'Why is God never unkind or wrong?' I tried, as well as I could, to explain the perfection of God's character. and its freedom from human frailties; but alas! how vain is the effort, when neither teacher nor pupil have any other standard than human littleness by which to measure God's greatness.

"There is this constant difficulty with her (and is it not one too much overlooked in the religious instruction of other children?), that being unable to form any idea of virtue and goodness in the abstract, she must seek it in the concrete; and her teachers and friends, frail and imperfect beings like herself, furnish the poor impersonations of the peerless attributes of God.

"This difficulty might have been avoided, I think, by the plan which I had marked out for the orderly development of her intellectual faculties and moral sentiments, and which was simply to follow the natural order; but since that plan has been marred by the well-meant officiousness of others, there remains only to remedy, as far as we can, what we cannot cure entirely —the bad effects of ill-timed direction of her thoughts to subjects too far above her comprehension.

"After the conversation related above, I went on to illustrate, as well as I could, the difference between human and divine care of animals. I said, 'Why does man take care of a cow, and get hay into his barn to feed her in winter?' 'Oh!' said she, 'to get her milk.' ' Why does he take care of his horse, and keep him covered with a warm blanket, and feed him?' ' That is to ride him well,' said she. ' Why do people keep cats, and feed them?' ' To catch mice.' ' Why do farmers take such good care of sheep?' ' To get wool.' ' But when the cow and the sheep are old, and cannot work, what does man do?' ' He kills to get meat.' ' Well,' said I, ' why does God make the grass to grow in the meadow, and let the cow eat it? Does he want her milk?' ' No,' said she. ' Does he need the wool of the sheep?' ' No!' replied she vehemently, ' he does not want anything.' Presently she said, ' How do men know whether cows are willing to give them their milk?' I said, ' They do not know and do not care.' She mused awhile, as is her wont when talking on a new subject, and said, ' The little lambs and young animals play : why do not sheep love to have their pleasure?' I explained how they had pleasure in giving milk to their young, how they loved to eat the tender grass, and lie in the shade. She seemed to have another difficulty, and said, ' Why do cats want to kill mice? They have no love!'' "

In closing the account of my stewardship, perhaps it will not be considered out of place for me to answer the question which has often been asked, and to which an answer ought to be given. It has been asked with great earnestness whether I think that Laura could have been made acquainted with the doctrines of the Bible at the time of my instructing her. I do suppose that she could have understood them, and my opinion is founded on the following reasons.

As soon as these doctrines were mentioned to her, she received them very readily. It was far more difficult to teach her many common things of life than to teach these truths, which indeed she learned so easily that we could not determine when and how she obtained her knowledge of them. Her soul seemed to be prepared for them, receptive of them. Very many of the questions, for answers to which I referred her to Dr. Howe, could have been answered without difficulty at the moment of her asking them. We could not divine where she acquired much of the knowledge she had; hints from the blind girls seemed to suffice as a clew, and then she worked out the rest herself.' She asked Dr. Howe, " What is a soul?" and received the idea at once. Could she not then have received the Biblical doctrines? A girl capable of asking such questions is capable of receiving the replies. It may be she could not receive them all clearly; neither did she receive all clearly in her other studies, but we did not delay the teaching on this account.

That the influence of my enforced reticence on such subjects was disastrous, may readily be perceived. While she entirely understood that it was the wish of Dr. Howe, and therefore refrained from asking me questions save when her soul was

so full it must find utterance, yet there was, especially in the last year of my intercourse with
her, an impatience in waiting that extended to
other things. Her mind was so full of these subjects that the most interesting lesson could not
exclude them, and as has been seen in the previous pages, when I supposed she was absorbed in
our conversation on other topics, she surprised me
with questions on religious topics, for replies to
which she must wait.

In another direction the bad effects were apparent. I was unable to appeal to the highest
motives. She was living under the old dispensa-
tion, and had not even the example of Christ as a
model ; for until my last month with her, she did
not even know his name.

Could Dr. Howe have anticipated her mental
development during his absence, he would doubtless have left her under the charge of some person who sympathized with his views and who
could have satisfied her questionings ; but it was
my privilege only to give the intellectual training
which should prepare the way for my more
favored successor.

I make these statements with no design to censure Dr. Howe, but merely to answer questions
regarding the difference of my opinions from those
entertained by that eminent philanthropist.

CHAPTER XV.

LAURA was without any regular instruction from the 1st of May until the last of August, 1845. At this time Miss Sarah Wight, who had taught several years in the girls' department of the Institution, took charge of her. For the report of the next few years we are indebted to her journal, which bears ample testimony to the faithfulness with which she discharged her onerous duties.

New arrangements were made by which Laura was kept constantly with her teacher, Dr. Howe having selected two or three of the blind girls, who were allowed to call upon her in her private room occasionally, for a play or chat.

By this means she was prevented from receiving any new ideas, except through the medium which he approved.

Miss Wight found that in the four months Laura had forgotten much with which she had been quite familiar, both in geography and arithmetic, which was not a matter of surprise.

From this time no records of the details of her lessons were kept, but we can judge of her intel-

lectual improvement from the evidence of it which
we find in the reports of conversation, and in the
extracts from her own journal. Miss Wight's
journal reports mainly her Bible study and the
development of her moral and religious character.

We make the following extracts : —

"One day, I remarked to her that the first settlers
of this country sometimes had difficulty in procuring
enough to eat ; whereupon she asked suddenly, 'What
repast did one man eat?' She explained herself by
adding, 'When there was but one man on the earth.'
The answer was that there was fruit and berries.
'But,' said she, 'when he was very small?' She
paused awhile, and then added, 'I guess God took
care of him, and gave him some milk.'

"I was reading something in which a compass was
mentioned ; upon which, she was desirous of knowing
all about it. I showed her a magnet, and applied it to
a toy in the shape of a swan floating upon the water.
When she felt that the bird was attracted by the magnet, her face grew very red, and she said, much surprised, 'It makes it live ; it is alive, for it moves.'
I then asked her if the bird ate or slept or walked or
could feel. 'No,' she replied, but still seemed hardly
convinced that the magnet did not give life to the bird,
until she was shown its effect upon a needle.

"This led to an explanation of attraction ; and she
soon afterwards showed her disposition to apply all new
words in as many senses as she can, by suddenly
embracing me and saying, 'I am exceedingly attracted
to you, because you are always so kind.'

"In one of our walks, after a long pause in the conversation, she asked me, while blushing and laughing,
'Do you think I shall ever be married with a gentleman whom I love best and most?' I said, 'No.
When she had thought of all the objections, she said,
'Mrs. Davis is married and she is blind. I can sweep
and fix things very nicely and do many things.'

" *Oct. 24.* At eight o'clock to-day Laura came to
me and said, 'Doctor wants you to teach me about
motives. What are motives?'

"After giving the meaning of the word, I referred her
to a story that I read to her last evening. It was of
a benevolent, kind-hearted little boy, who expended
his money in purchasing little comforts for those who
needed them, making it his happiness to do good to the
poor and unfortunate. She was very much interested
in talking of the character of the boy, and of his sister
and mother. It was a good motive for George to give
nice things to poor people. Doctor had a good motive
to give us this nice large room to be so warm and comfortable. He is very benevolent. But Jesus Christ
was the most benevolent; we cannot be benevolent as
he was. I cannot be benevolent and do kind things to
crazy people, and blind and deaf people, and cure them.
God is very benevolent, he does so many things to make
people happy. I then tried to show her how she might
be truly benevolent in little things, every day. 'I
give away many things,' said she. I convinced her
that it was not alway a proof of *benevolence* to give
things away. During the whole lesson she was very
serious and thoughtful, pressing my fingers closely, so
that no letter should escape her.

" *Oct. 25.* Laura seemed to me rude and boisterous, and not easily restrained as usual. It was very discouraging to me, and I gave myself up to sad thoughts. Laura soon perceived it, and asked why. I told her she did not try, so much as 1 wished, to grow still and gentle, though we had talked so much about it. She sat still some time, and then said, ' I love Mrs. Smith best, she is so gentle.' This was evidently said to trouble me, and did not relieve me any. This is one of the very few instances where there seemed to be unkindness in the child's heart. But she soon repented. After dinner she was up stairs, and was gone for some time ; when at last she came down and found me, she said she had a nice present for me to make me more happy, and that she would try more to improve. She said this very sadly. I took her present and exerted myself to appear as cheerful as usual. The present she brought was a pincushion, one of her choicest treasures.

" Lessons as usual. Talking with Laura about being kind and benevolent. She began to give me a long account of little kind things that she had done. After a time I told her that sometimes people did kind things that their friends might praise them and think they were very kind and benevolent. We talked of it some time, Laura's face growing more and more red, yet half smiling. 1 could see she was applying the remark to herself, as indeed she does everything that she hears of this kind. ' Why do I like to be praised?' she soon asked. I told her that every one did, and that it was right for us to like to have our friends love us, and praise us too, if we were good. Supposed the case of two little children, one of whom was very kind to his sisters that his mother might call him good, and the other did the same because he was glad to see all happy, etc. Asked her which she thought was the best child. She hesitated a moment, and replied, ' The boy who wanted to see other children happy '

" *Nov. 4.* Laura asked me, ' Why do I have two thoughts? Why do I not do what my conscience tells me is right?' Told her I thought when she began to do wrong she was in play, and afterwards her firmness led her to continue to do wrong, though her conscience was telling her all the time she was wrong.

" *Nov. 10.* Laura went to church with me in the morning. In the afternoon, I left Jane with her, with permission to stay a short time. When I returned, Laura did not welcome me as usual, and made some objection to a walk which I proposed; but she was soon ready for it. I learned from Jane that Laura had done something that she (Jane) had promised not to tell me. I asked Laura why she was not willing that I should know everything that she did while I was away. She said, ' I was afraid you would reprove me.' I asked her if I ever spoke unkindly to her when she had done wrong. ' No,' replied she, very emphatically, ' you never blame me. Why did I pull the wire?' I answered that I thought curiosity and playfulness made her do it; that it was not wrong to be curious and playful, but that it was wrong to try to conceal from me when she thought she had done mischief. ' I did not know it was to conceal,' said she. I told her that it was best for me to know what she did and thought, that I might be able to advise her. ' I knew it was wrong to pull the wire.' Jane had told me also that Laura was unwilling that she should leave her, and made several very unpleasant noises. I alluded to this when talking to Laura, and she said, ' I was not impatient.' ' But,' said I, ' Jane said you made some bad noises.' ' I did n—,' she began to say hesitatingly, when I said, ' Did you not make noises?' and she replied, ' I believe I did not refrain from making bad noises.' I was now obliged to leave her for a short time. When I came back, she was not inclined to say much, and seemed trying to force a smile. By this time, the head-ache which had followed me all day became quite severe, and I left her again for a while to her reflections. It is the first time that she has attempted to deceive me. She was afraid, perhaps, that she had done some injury to something. She could have no fear that I should speak severely to her, for I never blame her in the least. Generally, when she is doing or saying any little thing that I disapprove, I simply stop it at the time, and afterwards speak of the thing abstractly. She will apply my remarks to herself and to the circumstance, but without any unpleasant excitement of feeling, and she remembers them a long time.

" Many times she has said, ' I cannot be perfectly good, as Jesus Christ was.' I have told her that every one should try to be perfectly good, and never be willing to do wrong even in a little thing; explained to her that perhaps it was a desire to appear perfectly good which prompted her to conceal that which she was afraid was wrong.

" When I spoke to her again, she said, ' I was praying to God, and told him that I had been so wrong, and I asked him to forgive me and send me better thoughts,

I told him my motives were bad to conceal from you, and to tell you that I did not make impatient noises.' She then put her hand on my hot head and asked, ' What made it worse?' I answered, ' Sad thoughts.' She said, ' I am sorry you were detained from being happy by a sad circumstance. I have told God that I will not do so wrong again.'

" *Dec. 13.* A good lesson in arithmetic, but Laura was not in her usual spirits. I said nothing, hoping it would wear off. After breakfast I told her that she said last night that she felt unkindly towards me and asked if she knew the cause of it, and if I said anything that troubled her. ' No, I think it was because I did not refrain from bad thoughts.' ' Do you know what made your thoughts bad? Was it because I showed you how you shook my arm?' ' No, I think my conscience was bad.' ' Our consciences are never bad, they will never tell us to do what we know is wrong: did you not know it was wrong?' ' Yes, but I did not obey my conscience, and that was the reason that I slapped you.' A few moments after she said, ' I am too old to be reproved.' ' But you are not too old to do wrong.' ' My mind can reprove me,' was her reply. I said, ' You do not wish to injure your teacher: why do you not tell her that you are sorry that you struck her?' She smiled and made no reply. I left her for half an hour to her own thoughts, and on speaking to her again, asked of what she had been thinking. ' Praying to God, for he can help me best. I asked him to send me good thoughts.' She did not say this with her usual seriousness, but as if repeating words merely, and added, ' People told me always to ask God

to help me.' I said, ' You struck your teacher who is
always kind to you: are you not sorry?' No reply.
' Do you think your thoughts are all good and your
feelings all kind now?' Still no reply. Not liking to
force an unwilling expression of sorrow from her, by
depriving her of her lessons, and having often found
that showing her some mark of kindness, or allowing
her to do something for me, would completely subdue
her bad feelings, I allowed her to give some account of
the story read to her yesterday, and then to write in
her journal. She wrote, that ' On Friday night she
struck her teacher and that it was very unkind,' and
brought it to me. I then asked her again if she knew
that she had not told me she was sorry. She said,
' Yes, I was just going to tell you that I am sorry, and
that I have resolved to control myself. I shall never
strike you again, I am so earnest to have my excellent
teacher happy always. I hope you will not think of the
bad thing any more, for you are my best teacher.'
After dinner we did not stop as usual to speak to Mrs.
S., and she asked why. Told her it was better for
her to think than to talk, and besides my head ached
badly. When I spoke of my head, the poor child threw
her arms around my neck, and put her head on my
shoulder saying, ' I am so sorry that your head aches to
think so much about me. I promised Martha that I
would always be kind to you. Did I hurt you very
much?' It was really painful to see her distress, and
I did the best I could to soothe her.

'' *Dec. 15.* Laura was very much perplexed by very
simple things, and I was obliged to repeat a simple
question many times at the risk of losing my own

patience. When the difficulty was overcome, she said with a triumphant air, ' I have persevered in being good, I have not been impatient any.'

"*Dec. 24.* She said this morning, 'Last night I dreamed so strangely. I thought I was but fifteen years old and that I was very sick and was going to die. At last you and Doctor put me in the ground, and I was so happy to be in heaven : my soul was in heaven, but when you put the earth on me, it gave me life again. Who can tell me all about how I shall know when my breaths are going, and I am going to die? Did you go to see Adeline in Cambridge? She was dead and they put her body in a box and put her in the ground. Why do they put people in the ground?' Told her they could not use their bodies any longer ; but that only the worn-out bodies were buried. She sat thinking some time and then said, ' Our souls do not die when our bodies are dead.' We then talked about the importance of taking good care of our minds if they lasted so long, and trying to make them good and honest and kind. We know the necessity of taking good care of our bodies, though they do not last long, etc. She added, ' It is very solemn to think soberly about death, and how very good we ought to be.' Several times in the day she returned to the same subject. At one time she asked, ' Are you sure that heaven is much larger than this world?' and said, ' Mrs. C. told me all about heaven. She said it was much larger and wider and higher than this world, to make room for many souls. Do you know about it?' I answered that I did not know, but that God was kind and good to every one, and that if we were good we should be happy anywhere. With great apparent satisfaction she summed up the whole subject in these words, ' He is our *Father,*' and then asked, ' Why did Jesus come on the earth?' I told her that he came to tell us how much God loved us, and to teach us to become good. She said, ' He made many sacrifices for men, he was so kind.'

"Christmas morning she said, ' We ought to remember and think much about Christ to-day, how good he was,' etc.

" She has often amused herself during the past year by little exercises in composition. The following story, written during the absence of her teacher, will serve as a specimen of her use of language. The last sentence, though not grammatical, may be considered as the moral, and a very good moral of the whole.

THE GOOD-NATURED GIRL.

Lucy was nearly nine years old. She had excellent parents. She always did with alacrity what her mother requested her to do. She told Lucy when it was time for her to go to school; so Lucy ran and put on her bonnet and shawl, and then she went back to her mamma. She offered Lucy a basket containing some pie and cake for luncheon. And Lucy went precisely at school-time and when she got to the house she took her own seat and began to study diligently with all the children. And she always conformed to her teacher's wishes. In recess she took luncheon out of her basket, but she gave some of it to her mates. Lucy had some books with pictures and slate in her desk. When she went home she found that dinner was all ready. Afterwards her mother took her to take tea with her friends. Lucy was much delighted to play with her little cousins, Lucy and Helen; and they let her see their playthings. After tea Lucy was sorry to depart; and when she went to bed she thought she had made it pleasantly to all her friends with little joyful heart.

"*Jan. 1, 1846.* Laura was full of glee this morning. ' I am so very happy. I have resolved to be so good. I am so happy to be alive.' Yesterday I commenced teaching her a Bible history. It will be exceedingly difficult to give her an idea of the history recorded in the Old Testament without confusing all her ideas of right and wrong, justice and humanity."

In the latter part of February the journal speaks of her as having been "obedient, generous, and self-denying; at times a little irritable for a moment, but soon recovering herself," and again, "she has learned many new words and phrases, but has not done as much as I expected in school. I have frequently omitted lessons when she seemed too nervous to attend to them." She continued to fail in health, and in May went with Miss Wight to Philadelphia to visit her former teacher. She had voluntarily adopted a diet of bread and milk, to which she strictly confined herself at each of her three meals. No delicacies could tempt her, although it seemed to all her friends that she was rapidly growing weaker in consequence of her persistence. She was interested in meeting old friends and in making new acquaintances, but soon became weary and languid.

It was decided on her return from the South to try the effects of her native air, and she went with her teacher to her home in Hanover.

From the journal of her visit there, we quote the following : —

"Laura appears very amiable and attentive to every one's wants, and exerts herself to do everything in her power to add to my comfort and happiness. She sometimes asks me if she sets her brothers a good example. She evidently feels that she is an older sister.

"It was pleasant to see her with Mr. Tenny ; she seemed to have entire confidence in him. Each time he visited her she wished to go to the barn in quest of eggs as she was accustomed to do when a child. She took his hand and would go alone with him with a confidence I have rarely seen her manifest towards a gentleman. Though they never found any eggs, she never tired of the search.

"One day she said, ' I will write some new things for my brothers to make them more wise.' She wrote rapidly on a slate the following : ' I hope that you love God very much, for he is so kind always, who supplies us with such beautiful flowers, and many other things in the world I love him extremely much, he is so benevolent. You must exert yourselves to think of him, how good and kind he is, and that he loves all of his children and to have them do what he wishes them. We will all be very happy with him, if we are always good and right, as long as we live, always.'

"*August, 1846.* Laura said, ' I dreamed last night

19

that I must die. I was very much afraid.' I talked
with her until she became quite cheerful.

"*Sept. 1.* Talked with Laura about our mutual
dependence. Told her that God did not intend we
should think only of ourselves, because he had so made
us that we could not be comfortable and happy without
the assistance and sympathy of those about us. She
asked, ' Why did God make me if he knew I should
have so many faults?' I replied, I thought he wished
her to correct her faults, and enjoy a very happy life,
and asked her if she had not lived many happy hours.
' Yes.' ' And why are you not always happy?' ' I do
not always feel right and do right.'

"She has seemed very well and happy to-day. At
first she was unwilling to take the shower-bath (which
was a new thing to her), but I told her it was thought
good for her and I hoped she had courage enough to
endure the disagreeable feeling for a minute. She
laughed and said she was very brave, and went in resolutely. While we were walking she wished to tell me
some curious dreams she had had recently. ' I dreamed
I wrote a letter to God, and tried very hard to get
some one to carry it. I told him that I wanted to
come to visit him very much. I dreamed that I was in
heaven once, and saw God with my eyes.' "

She had been persuaded during the summer to
ride a little upon a donkey, and now overcame
her timidity sufficiently to mount a pony. She
rode frequently, having a person to accompany
her to hold the bridle, and enjoyed the exercise
very much.

" *Sept. 11.* After Laura's ride on the pony, took her to be weighed, and found her weight to be but seventy-nine pounds. She seemed a little troubled by it, and I told her I thought if she ate a little meat and some vegetables she would grow heavier and stronger also. ' I do not like meat,' was her reply. ' But will you not try to eat a little and learn to like it, if you do it only to please me?' ' No,' she replied with a most unamiable emphasis. I was no less surprised than grieved at such an answer, for heretofore, although she has frequently differed in opinion. she has been ready to yield to me. In all little things she obeys me without hesitation. or, ' with alacrity,' as she often says. She is too old for us to expect her to render the blind obedience of a child, but her self-esteem will make her unhappy in her future life unless checked now. Her situation has always been one adapted to strengthen this feeling. She has a seat apart from the other pupils in the school-room, and she knows that she is an object of more interest than any of the other blind girls."

During the autumn, with the return of cooler weather, her health improved and she resumed her lessons, and in December she was again at work in arithmetic, having advanced as far as Interest. She was also having lessons in grammar.

" *Dec. 23.* Rev. Dr. Wayland came to see Laura, and asked her many questions. He read a story which she had written, as easily, he said, as if he had written it himself. He asked if he might take a copy of it for his son, and she told him she would send it to him for a Christmas present. Before leaving the doctor gave her money to purchase a Christmas present for herself. She decided that it would give her more pleasure to expend it in the purchase of presents for her friends. The afternoon was spent in the selection of presents. Among others she remembered a little girl who was sick, Lizzie who was deaf, Mrs. C.'s little girl who was lame. There is nothing more beautiful in Laura's character than the love and pity she shows for all the afflicted, however uninteresting they may be in other respects. When she met poor Harriet, the negro, she shrank from the touch of her hand, 'it was so bony and strange,' but when she knew that she was sick, she would remind me to go and see her, and was anxious that I should do everything I could for her, and herself bought nice fruit to send her.

"*Dec. 30.* In our walk to-day I checked her when she was making one of her noises. She asked if I remembered when she used to be impatient when she was told not to make a noise; she said, 'I used to be impatient and look cross and say unkind things. I can be good and gentle so much easier than I could a year ago.' I replied, 'We are a great deal happier now, that we do not have such things to trouble us.' And she said, 'I hope this (new) year we shall not have one unkind, wrong thing to make us unhappy.' Told her I thought she had improved much and hoped she would improve as much next year. 'Yes, more,' was her reply. She asked to-day, 'How can I became distinguished?'"

At the close of the year 1846, Dr. Howe writes : —

" It was stated in the report of Laura Bridgman, which was made in January last, that her health had been failing during several months, and was then very feeble. I am sorry to say that it continued to grow weaker for some time, and has not yet become entirely re-established.

'' During most of the past year she has been weak and sickly. In the spring especially, she became very much emaciated, her appetite failed almost entirely, and she could hardly be persuaded to take nourishment enough to keep her alive.

'' She was placid and uncomplaining, and though never gay as in former years, she was never gloomy. She appeared to feel no fear or anxiety concerning her health, and when questioned closely about it she would answer that she was very well. Indeed, the change had come over her so slowly and gradually that she seemed to be hardly conscious of it, and showed surprise when it was alluded to. Sometimes, indeed, when she found that she was wearied by walking half a mile, she was forced to remember her former long walks of five and six miles, and to think about the change.

'' As she grew thinner and paler and weaker, she appeared to be laying aside the garments of the flesh, and her spirit shone out brighter though its transparent veil. Her countenance became more spiritualized, and its pensive expression told truly that, though there was no gloom, neither was there any gladness in the heart.

'' Her intellect was clear and active, and she would fain have indulged in conversation and study about subjects of a serious nature ; but she was sensitive and excitable, and the mental activity and craving were

perhaps morbid. Be that as it may, however, she was
at a fearful crisis in her life, and it seemed to be our
first duty to save that. She was therefore not only
diverted from all exciting trains of thought, but dis-
suaded from pursuing her usual course of study. We
were very desirous not to alarm her by showing the
anxiety which was really felt about her; and this object
was gained so effectually that she probably did not
discover her danger. She is always very observant,
however, and ascertains the state of mind of those about
her by reading parts of the natural language of the
emotions, which we never observe, but which are as
sure guides to her as the expression of the countenance
is to us. It is almost impossible that her companions
should feel particularly gay or sad, and withhold the
knowledge of it from Laura. The natural language of
the feelings is almost infinite. A common observer
reads only the page of the countenance, the keener one
finds meaning in tones of the voice, or, looking more
closely, reads signs in the very shaking of hands; but
Laura not only observes the *tones of the finger language*,
she finds meaning in every posture of the body and in
every movement of limb; in the various play of the
muscles she observes the gentle pressure of affection,
the winning force of persuasion, the firm motion of
command, the quick jerk of impatience, the sudden
spasm of temper, and many other variations which she
interprets swiftly and correctly.

    " With all these means of ascertaining the state of
her teacher's feelings, and with the certainty that an
untrue answer would never be given her, Laura would
surely have learned that her life was thought to be in ·

some danger if she had ever been accustomed to dwell upon thoughts of sickness and death ; but she had not, and therefore she walked without a shudder upon the brink of the grave.

" The result was as I had hoped and expected that it would be, for I was more sanguine than others. The natural strength of her constitution, which had triumphed in that fearful struggle during her infancy, though at the expense of two of the most important organs of sense, had been carefully nurtured by constant exercise, simple diet, and regular habits of mind and body, and it carried her safely through this second trial. After she had been brought so low that it seemed as if the tendency to disease could find no more resistance to overcome, it yielded at last, and then the vital powers began to rally slowly.

" When the weather grew warmer, she began a course of sea-bathing and of exercise upon horseback. These occupied and amused her mind and strengthened her body ; and she continued to grow better through the year, very slowly, indeed, but surely. She has now recovered some portion of her lost flesh ; and her appetite is so far restored that she eats a sufficient quantity of bread and milk, but does not like anything else. She does not wish to change her food at all, but when meal-time arrives, she sits down cheerfully to her simple bread and milk, morning, noon, and evening, and having finished that, she disregards all the dainties and the fruits with which the capricious appetite of invalids is usually tempted. Her present diet is one of her own choice, and though it is not the best, and its sameness is unwise, we do not insist upon a change while she is

manifestly thriving, because it might do more harm
than to indulge a caprice of appetite, not uncommon
with delicate persons.

" But the best sign of returning health is the change
which has taken place in her animal spirits, nor is this
change uninteresting in a moral point of view. Before
her illness, she was not only a happy, but a merry child,
who tripped cheerfully along her dark and silent path
of life, bearing sportfully a burden of infirmity that
would have crushed a stout man, and regarding her
existence as a boon given in love, and to be expended
in joy ; since her illness, she seems to be a thoughtful
girl, from whom the spontaneous joy of childhood has
departed, and who is cheerful or sad in sympathy with
the feelings of those about her.

" I hope and believe that her health will be perfectly
restored, although it is still very frail, and easily de-
ranged by any over-exertion of body or mind. Perhaps a complete change may take place in her physical
system, and her now slender form develop itself into
the proportions of a large woman ; such changes are
not unfrequent after such severe crises. At all events,
with restoration of health will come a return to those
studies and occupations which have been necessarily
suspended.

" She was just beginning to understand that, as she
was getting freed from her obligations of unconditional
obedience to those who had directed her childhood, she
must come under no less unconditional obedience to the
new monitor and master, the conscience, that was as-
serting its rule within her ; and the veneration and
affection for human friends, which are the first objects

of the awakened germ of the religious feeling, were gradually tending upwards and expanding into worship and love of God.

" This transformation of her soul, this disinthral-ment of its high and independent powers, was becom-ing perfectly clear to her by means of instruction, and would have changed what had been mere habit and blind obedience into conscious duty and stern principle, but the process was necessarily interrupted. Such in-struction would of course require the consideration of subjects which were to her of the most intensely excit-ing interest, and might have cost her life.

" I know that many will say that I had already com-mitted a great error by deferring the consideration of these subjects so long, and that I should have tried to retrieve it by giving at once the knowledge which they suppose necessary to eternal salvation, even at the ex-pense of mortal life. To this I have only to answer, that I have gratefully received and carefully weighed all the counsel which has been given to me in the spirit of kindness, but that it has failed to alter my views of my duty.

" A general review of her character and deportment during the past year gives rise to some agreeable reflec-tions. In former years, though she presented an ex-traordinary example of gentleness, truthfulness, and affection, she showed, like most children, occasional ex-cesses of feeling, which required her conduct to be under the regulation of others, so that she was not entirely a free moral agent. During the last year the reins of authority have been slackened ; she has been allowed to follow more freely her own inclinations, and though her

teacher has been, as in former years, her constant companion, and doubtless exercised great influence over her,
yet her society and companionship have been rather
sought by Laura than imposed upon her. Opportunity
has thus been given her to develop her individuality of
character, and to exercise her moral powers by self-
guidance.

" It would have been practicable to keep her in leading-
strings still longer, and by taking advantage of habit,
to require unconditional obedience for years to come,
though this might have been difficult, for she evidently
inherits a strong self-will ; but the time had arrived when
she ought to begin to govern herself ; she showed considerable capacity for doing so, and it would have been
wrong to keep her in subjection.

" Not only was it right to give her considerable freedom of action, but to have withheld it would have been
injurious to her moral growth, by the loss of that exercise in self-government which prepares one for complete
independence of thought and action. The result of
leaving her in comparative freedom has shown that self-
government, when the proper age for it has arrived, and
the previous habits have been good, is as much better
than foreign government, as walking by the aid of its
own bones and muscles is better for a child than going
in leading-strings.

" Her thoughts, as I remarked before, have been of a
more serious nature, and her conduct more sober, during
the past year, than in former times. This is probably the
natural consequence of the lowered tone of her physical
health, and not, as I have been able to discover, of any
thought or fear of death.

" Already with returning health and strength there appear glimpses of her former gayety of heart; and though she may never again be the merry, thoughtless girl that she was, we may hope to see in her a happy and cheerful woman. She will no longer be the same object of public curiosity and interest that she has been, but she will not be the object of less care and affection to her friends so long as her frail life shall last."

CHAPTER XVI.

THE only record of the year 1847, we find in Miss Wight's journal, extending through the first six months. We select the following entries : —

"*Jan. 4, 1847.* Laura said she should like to be excused from the shower-bath on Sunday as she wanted more time. She wished she had a Bible to read in herself. I told her I could read to her from mine. She replied, ' But it is much better to read the Bible ourselves.' I soon convinced her that she could not understand it if she should attempt to read it alone, and she said, ' I wish you would read to me every day in the Bible. How did God tell the first man about himself?' Told her I did not know exactly, but that God gave men minds capable of thinking of him, and some very good men had many thoughts about God. She asked, ' And did they tell each other and each other, so that all the young children might know about God?' 1 added that at last Christ came, and he told the people much more about God. ' How long has God lived?' My answer puzzled her apparently. She sat holding my hand while thinking ; she was trying to grasp infinity, and then asked, ' Why can we not think how *very* long God has lived?'

' *Jan. 5.* It was a bright, warm day, and as we walked ⸺aura stopped and turned her face upward toward the sun, saying, ' It is very pleasant. Why does our heavenly Father let his sun shine on us in our wrong days? ' I do not know why she spoke of wrong days, unless because. half an hour before, she told me half impatiently that I spelled a word incorrectly. Of late she has not shown any of those little impatient feelings that we used to see so much when everything was not as she wished it. It is seldom now that she gives me one troubled thought. It seems as if she had no wrong thoughts, for she certainly does not express them in look, word, or act. She has seemed more quietly happy than I have ever known her before.

'' *Jan. 10.* Laura asked me as usual about the sermons that I had heard during the day, The subject of the afternoon was ' forgiveness.' On hearing this, her first eager inquiry was, ' How can I know if God has forgiven me, for I used to do wrong so often? ' I gave her an account of the sermon, which seemed to satisfy her.

'' *Jan. 14.* At noon commenced reading the second chapter of Matthew to Laura. The first eight verses occupied us closely for more than half an hour. She asked question upon question At last she began to grow nervous, and I took her to the school-room to divert her mind. She said as I closed the book, ' We shall be so happy to meet Christ when we go to heaven. I wish we could see him now here with us.'

'' *Jan. 15.* Finished reading the second chapter of Matthew. Laura was shocked at the perfidy of Herod in pretending that he wished to worship Christ, when

he wished to destroy him, and with his cruelty in order-
ing the destruction of the infant children of Bethlehem ;
she was much afraid that Herod would at last discover
where the infant Jesus had gone.

"*Jan. 18.* She asked to hear again the chapter that
I had read, and in addition I read the account of
Christ's visit to Jerusalem at the age of twelve years
as recorded in Luke. She asked if he did right to
stay away from his parents to make them sorrowful.

"*Jan. 29.* Gave her a copy of the New Testament
that she might read herself the fifth chapter of Matthew. It is a very slow process, for every sentence
must be explained. Almost every day when I have
been explaining something, she tells me, ' Yes, I knew
before ; you have told me many times.' Though she
knows little of the form in which the Scriptures are
written, she is familiar with their spirit. She was interested in the blessing promised to the pure in heart.
When I had told her what was meant by seeing God,
and that the pure and good were more like God,
could understand his character better, would think of
him more, and love him better, she asked, ' Is God
near our minds? Could we be as happy if he was not
with us? How do you know we could not live without him?' She read over two or three times, ' Ye are
the salt of the earth.' She asked, ' What did Christ
mean? We are not salt.'

"*Feb. 1.* Laura received a letter from her mother
containing intelligence of the death of her old friend,
Mr. Tenny. As I read the letter her face was first
red and then turned pale again. She said, ' I am very
sad that my oldest friend is dead, that I never can see

him again. But I think he is much happier now, for he was always so good and kind to everybody. She sat by me in silence, and then said half inquiringly, ' I think Mr Tenny can see us now.' She called to mind the many little kindnesses the poor old man had shown her, and thought of nothing else until she prepared to go to church with me. She had a crape badge which had been worn at the time of President Harrison's death, and wished to wear it

" *Feb. 3.* Laura still thinks much of Mr Tenny. His death has sensibly affected her. Beside her regret for him, she feels the reality of death more than ever before. She asked, ' Do you think I shall be afraid when I am dying? I do not understand how people feel when they are dying.'

" *Feb. 6.* I read and explained the Lord's Prayer. After this she wanted me to tell her about prayer, how we could pray, etc. I told her that we prayed for those things that we desired most earnestly to receive, and asked her what she thought we needed most, and should be most anxious to receive. Her reply was, ' To be sorry when we have done wrong, and for God to forgive us.' ' Do you think of anything else?' ' Goodness,' she added with emphasis.

" *Feb. 8.* Laura went to church with me, and asked the subject of the sermon. I told her, Christ's temptations. She said, ' Christ was never tempted to do wrong ! It is not true, I cannot credit it.'

" *Feb. 12.* She went to a dentist to have a tooth extracted, and attempted to take ether to produce insensibility to pain, but she was much alarmed when she perceived that it was depriving her of the power of

motion and of thought; she fancied she was dying, and
said she dreamed of God and heaven while she was
without the power of motion.   It was finally decided to
take it out without the gas, and she bore it bravely.

"*Feb. 14.*   She wrote to her brother to-day, ' Do
you like to endeavor to imitate Christ?   Christ was
very perfect, & had such a very beautiful character.
My dearest teacher Wight teaches me six lessons every
day. arithmetic, history, Bible & reading stories,
grammar & writing journal, & other different things.
I like to hear of Christ & his character, & our
Father, the best of all in the world.   Do you both learn
to comprehend the Bible much better than last summer?
I should like you to write to me all about your imitating Christ.   I am very sad not to see my oldest &
dearest friend, Mr. Tenny, ever on this earth.   I used
to love & respect him very much.   When I am in
Hanover again I should miss him.   It would appear
very lonely to me also.   I have the pin which he gave
me when I visited you all.   I used to wear it every day,
& remember him by it constantly.   Where is his body
buried?'

"*Feb. 16.*   Dr. Howe spoke to-day of the improvement in Laura's character that has taken place the last
year.   This may be ascribed in part to the quiet life
that she has led, and in part to the rule that I have
always observed, of never allowing even the slightest
fault to pass without some notice, at the time or afterward.   She has learned ' that it is more blessed to give
than to receive,' for she is evidently more pleased when
she can bestow a present than when she receives one.
Another reason for her improvement may perhaps be

found in a remark she made to me the last time she manifested any impatience. ' I thought quickly about Jesus Christ, how good he was, and then my good feelings came again.'

" *March 24.* To-day, for the first time, she seemed to be struck with wonder at the account of the miracles recorded as performed by Christ. Before this time she received all as a matter of fact, but to-day in reading the eighth chapter of Matthew she asked, ' How did Christ heal the sick? Did he give them medicine? How could they get well so quickly? ' I replied that I could not tell how, that some good people thought that Matthew was mistaken, but that Christ was so much purer and better than any one else, he might have power that we do not know of. This seemed to satisfy her. Her implicit faith in what she is told makes me tremble lest I should mislead her. ' If Christ had been here when Jane Damon was sick, do you think he would have cured her? Would he have cured me when I was sick, so that I should not have been deaf and blind? ' I tried to show her how Christ would do much more for us now than to cure our sickness of body, if we loved his character and tried to imitate it.

" *April 1.* Laura asked, ' Why did God make us to be sick and suffer pain if he loved us? ' I reminded her of the pain she had suffered from a slight burn, and told her that this pain might have saved her from much greater injury. Then we talked of the various ways in which life might be saved by attending to the warning that speaks to us so loudly through physical suffering ; of the effects of eating improper food, of neglecting exercise, bathing, exposure to cold air, etc.

20

"*April 2.* While Laura was reading, I asked her to repeat twice a word that she had spelled incorrectly, and that I did not understand. She seized my hand and in her impatience put my finger between her teeth as if she would have bitten it, but suddenly recollecting herself, she kissed it and turned away her face, which, from being pale, became very red. In an instant she turned to me, saying, ' Will you please to forgive me, for I shall never do such a thing again. It is so natural for all people to be impatient sometimes, except some very kind people who **are** never impatient. I think they try to imitate Christ. I feel impatient in my mind sometimes, but I do not let you know it.' I told her that probably every one felt it sometimes, but when we had learned to control the expression of it, the feeling could not last long. 'Are you ever impatient? But you never let your impatience act.'

"*Easter Sunday.* Talking of the sermon that I had heard, I was led for the first time to speak to Laura of the manner of Christ's death. 'Were the people not very unkind? Why did not Christ escape?' were her questions. Tried to show her how Christ had manifested his love for men by persisting in teaching the truth, though he knew that the end of it must be a cruel death; also that while Christ lived his disciples hoped that he would help them to be free from the Romans, and that it was only after his ignominious death that they could realize that he was a teacher, and not a governor.

"*April 4.* We read, ' But if ye forgive not men their trespasses, neither will you Heavenly Father forgive you.' She said, ' But I am sure our benevolent Father will forgive us if we do not forgive others.' This led to a long conversation on the subject of forgiveness, in what it consists, etc. She said, ' We shall be with God when we die.' ' Yes.' ' But heaven is an immense place, much larger than this earth, for one of my friends told me so many years ago.' She clings to this idea of a place of habitation for happy spirits. 1 convinced her that the situation in which we were placed did not of itself make us happy or miserable, by appealing to her own experience and that of others around her. She asked, ' How can I be sure that God is always with us?'

" *May 1*. Dr. Howe has decided to take Laura's religious instruction entirely into his own hands. She returned from her lesson to-day very eager to talk with me. ' Doctor says I must remember when I read the Bible that there are many mistakes in it. Do you believe there is any revelation? Doctor says some people do not believe it, but there surely is. Why do you not teach me as Doctor does about the Bible?' I replied that we did not think exactly alike about all things. ' Why not?' she asked, and seemed a little troubled. Her color changed and she looked very serious for a few moments, and then said, ' Why is your manner more diffident and timid than Doctor's when you talk to me about God and the Bible? And when you talk about wrong things you speak more gently and sadly, and not so firmly, as other people do.'

" *June 1*. We left Boston for a visit to Hanover, and met Laura's father in Concord. In the course of the journey she made many inquiries about her old friend, Mr. Tenny. She asked me, ' Would you like to go with me to see the place where he was buried, for

I should like to go? Do you think he was sad not to
see me again before he died? I shall miss him constantly. Do you think he can see us now, and know
what we are thinking about?' I tried to give her
pleasant thoughts and told her that her friend, who
was so kind to her, was not in the ground, that he
was still living, more loving than ever, and much happier than when he was in his poor sick body. Again
she asked, ' How can I know when I am going to die?'
and with a shudder said, ' I hope I shall not be sick.'
I talked quietly and gently with her of God's love and
care for all things he had made ; told her how He took
care of the birds and the bees, and all living things, and
how sure we might be that he would do all that was
best for us. She grew calm and even cheerful by
degrees. I do not intend to talk with her now on such
subjects, but under such circumstances it was unavoid-
able. In the course of the conversation she said,
' Heaven is above us over the sky. Can you see into
heaven? Look, up—up.' I told her, ' We were in
heaven now, when we were good and doing good.'
' And about the bad? How will God prevent the bad
from going to heaven?' I replied that those who had
bad feelings could not be happy anywhere, and convinced her that no place or circumstances could make
her happy, if she were conscious of doing or desiring
any wrong thing.

" Mr. Tenny remembered her to the last, and only
a few weeks before his death he tried to write to her, but
was unable to finish the letter. A day or two before he
died he wished that he had money to buy a basket of
an Indian woman for the deaf, dumb, and blind child.

" Almost all the pleasant remembrances which Laura has of the first part of her life seem to be associated with Uncle Asa, as he was familiarly known through the village. While her mother was absorbed in her household duties, he carried or led her gently from one neighbor's to another ; over the hills in search of berries and nuts ; to the fields for apples ; to the barn for eggs ; to the brook to show her the running water ; in short, he seemed to have found his happiness in trying to amuse this afflicted child.

" The sight of Laura seems to recall him to the minds of all the people, and almost every one has some story to tell of ' the time when she was a little thing, and came to see them with Uncle Asa.'

" *June 29.* We returned from Hanover to Boston. Laura enjoyed her visit very much, but made her preparations for leaving with great cheerfulness.

" *July 11.* Laura remained at home writing. After church I found her unusually nervous, even sad. Yesterday, as well as to-day, her mind has been full of thoughts of sickness, of death, of heaven, etc. For every one whom she meets she has a question ready. This seems to me unfortunate for her, as she is now I am afraid this uncomfortable state of mind has been brought on in part by the change which she has probably noticed in me. I have rather avoided such subjects instead of talking freely and naturally as formerly with her. I am sure it is best for Laura to be with one whose thoughts and feelings are so nearly right that the child can feel that they are not intentionally concealed from her. I am sure that Dr. Howe can teach her infinitely better than I can, yet important as his instructions may be to her, they cannot take the place of the words that she craves daily and hourly from a friend who is constantly with her. It is almost overwhelming when one thinks of all that is needed for the judicious training of one child, so much wisdom and so much goodness!

"*July 12.* Doctor tells me it is better that I should answer her questions upon all subjects, and not try to avoid conversing with her on any.

"*July 13.* Laura's lesson in history was upon Thebes. She expressed her surprise that the people were so fond of fighting. 'Did the Thebans and Spartans and Persians know about our Father? I do not think they did, for they would not fight so much.' When speaking of God now she always says 'our Father.' When we talk of a beautiful flower, a pleasant day, a little infant, or anything that interests her, it is not uncommon for her to ask, 'Does it remind you of our kind Father in heaven?' She asked, 'Are there any people on the earth who are afraid to leave their bodies?' I reminded her again of that part of Christ's teachings that interested her so much when she read it, of God's care even for the sparrows. She asked, 'How long shall you live? I shall be very sad when you die.' 'Why did God clothe our spirits with flesh? Why did he give us eyes and ears and hands? I want to read the Psalms, I can understand them so much better now. I wish you would resume your reading to me in the Bible, it makes me the happiest to know about Christ and God. I am very happy now, much happier than three years ago. I thank you very much for your good influence on me.'

"Talking one day about the ancient Greeks, she

said, ' I am glad we are so much better and happier than
barbarians. We shall be much happier in heaven.'

" I have observed several times of late a feeling of
satisfaction with herself at her own improvement. I
have tried to remove this in part by giving her examples of the greatest goodness and excellence, that she
may feel that there is yet something above her that she
may attain, but her natural self-esteem, joined to the
consciousness of possessing many right and kind feelings, often fills her heart with thankfulness that she is
' not as other men are.' "

" Let him that thinketh he standeth take heed
lest he fall," was verified in Laura's case, for after
months of exemption, she yielded again on two or
three occasions to her besetting sin of anger, only,
however, to reach greater depths of penitence, and
to make new resolves never to be overcome again.

From July, 1847, we find no notes by Miss
Wight until October, 1847, but fill the gap by
extracts from Laura's own journal, which she was
in the habit of writing daily.

Under date of Jan. 6, 1848, after noting the
occupations of the morning, she writes : —

" In the P. M. we had a pleasant conversation for
a while. As Miss W. was talking to me very kindly, I
was so reckless as to disobey my best impulse. I felt
an impatient feeling in my heart which made me wring
my poor teacher's delicate hand. At last she left me
alone. I took my work to occupy myself. I meditated

upon Christ who accomplished much good for every one. I now owned that I had done wrong. At length I went to W. & kissed her, for her to know how sad I felt; I assured her that I would exert myself to cultivate patience, & not have such bad feelings in the future. She was very kind to soothe me. I finished the basket, & then she taught me two lessons as usual."

She knew that her journal was read by Dr. Howe, but although always ambitious to appear well to him, and to do nothing to incur his disapprobation, she does not accompany this simple story of her fault by one word of extenuation. In this she was certainly superior to most children.

At this time a little girl totally deaf and partially blind was a member of the school, and as much of her instruction was given by the finger alphabet, it was thought that it might be well for Laura to have an opportunity to help some one, and so she was appointed her teacher for an hour a day. How she performed the duties of her new office will be seen from her own reports.

"*Jan. 19.* I instructed Lizzie a lesson from arithmetic with much pleasure. It seemed very funny and queer that I could teach a pupil so successfully."

This was probably her first lesson. One day she wrote, —

"When I was teaching her very earnestly, she mentioned that she wished to have sport so much, but I

Insisted upon her studying till the recess arrived. She conversed with me about her comical dreams of Miss W. & I & her mother."

Again, —

" As I spoke to my favorite pupil she would not reply to me, for she did not have a pleasant feeling in her own heart. It appeared to me that she did not feel inclined to have her lesson at first, but in a little time she was evidently willing to recite her lesson to me."

Another entry is, —

" At twelve I instructed my dear pupil. As I approached her, she denoted a very sweet and earnest expression upon her countenance to me, and it gratified my heart much."

Still another is, —

" As I approached my little pupil she did not feel inclined to be studious and diligent. I taught her about England for a while. When I mentioned to her that Miss W. considered that it would be the best plan for me to teach her a lesson in arithmetic, she said eagerly that I had promised to teach her geography. Lizzy was discontented & disappointed that I delayed teaching her geography."

Her journal entry for Feb. 25 is copied entire. It is the only time in which she speaks of her private devotions.

" Maria came & entered to call me. As soon as I rose, I delayed the shower-bath, for the room seemed excessively cold so that I felt a little apprehensive of being frozen. After I was thoroughly dressed I came into our tranquil parlour before I took my prayer. I took the precaution of locking the door, so that no one could come in to annoy me during my prayer. I knelt down by a chair to pray to God. I recited my lessons very diligently. At ten I taught my favorite pupil Lizzy a lesson in arithmetic, she appeared much more attentive and studious than usual in my opinion. After her lesson I communicated to her about my heavenly Father, with much pleasure and anxiety. She loved to make many inquiries of me about him I have had a very pleasant meditation. I thought much about God constantly; that when I do a sin in the least, my heavenly Father is tormented & disapproves of me, & likewise rebukes me for doing an error. When I am doing any thing wrong he remonstrate(s) or warn(s) with me. When I think of him I feel as though that he would forgive me, & send me a pure loving heart and happiness; then I feel reverent, & love him. When I am released from my body, I should be much happier to be with God forever, than on earth. I should love to see his best son Christ with him incessantly. I shall be much wiser and better when I die, than I am in the world. When I think of him, it causes me to have much happiness, & love, & to have the best of feelings, and reflections, & impulses, & qualities, & to do the duty of my heavenly Father."

She reports insubordination of her pupil and its punishment.

" *March 1.* I taught Lizzy a lesson at ten o'clock. She studied very industriously for a while. She then became so sportive that I was compelled to defer my instruction. As I assured Miss W. that L. said that she should not study, Miss W. considered that L. had better sit silently, for she was not faithful and innocent. I was obliged to read in my book by myself. I was very sorry to deprive L. of her long lesson."

The unceasing care and attention bestowed on Laura had so prostrated Miss Wight that she was obliged to leave her for a rest of some weeks. In her entry May 11, Laura writes a very tender and loving tribute to her.

" I thought if W. had a whole vacation as regularly as the (other) teachers & their pupils do, then she would regain her health & strength, so that she could have such a good resolution to instruct me much. I am sorry & anxious that she should have a vacation every time the other people do. It is likely that she would have enjoyed her instruction much afterwards. I do not trust (suppose) that she would have so perfect health, & so much strength as myself, for it is very unnatural to her. She can be very calm & cheerful instead of manifesting her activity & gayety: but I cannot tell how she looks in her sweet countenance. I wish I could discern her expression. I am willing that she should be sedate & much less emphatic, but I love to caress her very much indeed. My heavenly Father was so very kind to give me such a nice, beautiful friend, who has a very warm, affectionate, loving, humble, sociable, sympathizing heart. I should love to have her visit me as frequently as she could, when we are separated from each other."

She writes, —

July 10. " I made many inquiries of W. about the Lord and his only beloved Son. I cannot be as perfect as the Lord, because it is impossible for anybody to imitate (equal?) him. I should be the happiest if I could strive to do as much good to every one as possible, when I am 20ty years old. I am extremely hopeful that my heart or mind will retain much love, & benevolence, & confidence, & faith, as long as I live. I should feel in my own heart that God was pleased to see how much I could strive to do the volition of him. I fear that I could not bear so much, when any one should be much vexed or irritable to me. How could I make them feel better and happier? I should make an effort to comfort them by my patience & smiles. If they would not submit to follow my best example, or appreciate my character (intentions) for some time, I should not know what I could do. How could I acquire the art of making them cultivate their humility & patience? It is very likely that they might cultivate them by seeing how patient & smiling I should be. I hope that I shall not be likely to find any one who is unkind, & too hard-hearted and prejudiced against me. I could not utter (speak) to them or talk with them with my own fingers. I could not teach any ignorant people about goodness & love & humility, &c.

" *Aug. 3.* Miss W. ceased to instruct me at quarter past 2 o'clock because I hit her face & also pinched her

thumb backward. I was a very wrong and unjust
scholar to hurt her so much. I did not obey my best
impulse, which was so very good not to allow me to do
two wrong things I was exceedingly abashed, & guilty
in my own heart. I felt that God had inflicted a great
punishment upon me. It made me feel much ashamed &
alarmed. I was afraid because I was so very (wrong) to
disregard God, who was much displeased to see my bad
feelings. He was very angry to see me do very wrong.
My conscience was very great and strong; it kept
reproaching me for many hours. I have been thinking
much of God who was right & merciful to punish me
for doing wrong. My poor heart was overwhelmed
& tormented all day. When I repented much, my
heart felt that God would forgive me much more than
Miss W. could. I am very hopeful that I shall not be
likely to do her any harm so long as she is with me. I
am so much ashamed & sad that I should do very wrong
in the sight of W. She cannot trust me that I shall
strive to cultivate patience & love as long as I live. I
did not mean to hurt my lovely teacher so many times
while I was her scholar. God can do me much good
himself. He can forgive me more than any one."

A day or two later she writes, —

" I have been thinking about our only creator, who
made the earth, sun, animals, fruits, &c., which are very
wonderful to us all. I am very glad that my mind was
made to live forever in heaven with God. Why was it
not made to die as the body?

" *Aug.* 7. I have been thinking of God & Christ
this P. M. I am highly delighted that God sent Christ

to reside on the earth, so that he might communicate many things to all the people. He was very religious to command the people to do right, & to do so much good to all. I cannot realize that Christ lived on the earth to do the will of God. I shall have reverence toward God, if I think as much as it is possible of him. I feel in my own heart that he is coming to see me from heaven, when I am thinking so earnestly of him. It helps my heart to have much love & respect for him. I hope to love & respect him the more & more as long as my life. It is impossible for me to appreciate his character & his only beloved son. I love to think of him so very much better than anything else. I am extremely glad to know that he cannot forsake me, & that he can love me much more than I can love him. I ought to be very grateful to him who is so kind to chastise me for a sin, for he loves to do me good. I cannot conceive how much mercy, & love, & kindness he has, because he is so very perfect.

" *Aug. 11.* There is a very poor woman who has lost her husband. She has four or five children. They are not all very well. Her husband was working beneath the earth a few weeks; who (he) was terribly hurt by the falling of the earth. The earth broke very suddenly, that hurt some of the laborers exceedingly indeed. I have much compassion upon the poor woman and her children. I am fearful that they have a scanty food or clothes. I rejoice much that it is so very warm that they do not need much clothing. I say to myself, if it was a cold season then the poor family would have suffered very much from the cold & storm. How could the woman procure some wood to make a large fire.

& a plenty of new clothes to protect her children from the cold? I suppose that some benevolent people would be very charming & bountiful, to give the poor so many necessaries as they could. I am grateful & happy that we have such quantity of food, & a great supply of clothes here. My heavenly Father is the most benevolent of any one in the world, who bestows everything upon us continually. I cannot conceive how very benevolent & kind he is, in my life."

Occasionally she indulged in pleasant anticipations both for herself and her teacher. Aug. 23 she writes, —

" This P. M. I have been thinking about Miss Wight & her little nice house. I shall be very hopeful that she will have a very nice house in her life. I cannot imagine who can console her whilst she dwells in her tiny house. If I should fulfil my promise in residing with her, I could give her all my aid. I could help her wash & wipe & put away all her dishes so very nicely. I could sweep my little chamber, & dust & fix it very nicely every day. I should love to assist her to select all the necessaries, much light furnishture, & many nice delicate dishes. She would have some small cups for the very best."

Another day her anticipations are not so bright; she writes, —

" Who could have all of my precious things when I die? I may probably have many new friends as long as I live. I hope that they would endear themselves to me by love, kindness & benevolence. I **cannot** imagine how much I could love & respect them. Could it not be very (in)convenient for them to make the letters with their fingers? Could they have as much time to converse with me as my old friends now? Could I anticipate much pleasure, & that I should be so very sociable & happy, & contented, & loving, when I lose all of my old friends? I should really mourn, & miss many of my very dear old friends very much.

" *Sept.* 7. I have been thinking about my mother & brother A. I wish that I could dine with them to-day. I could probably have a better appetite with my dear family. We should find at mother's house a great profusion of pies & pumpkins & squashes & baked sweet apples & other nice victuals."

Occasionally she indulged in jokes, as in the entry for Jan. 19, 1849. She says, —

" I think that the rat ought to be imprisoned for stealing my beautiful apple the other day. He ought to have a conscience on purpose to reprove himself very much. I must ask W. to please to teach him about doing right & wrong & (being) honest in the night. He would love her very much for her good influence. She must exert herself to devote her time to instruct the rat about goodness, etc."

CHAPTER XVII.

AFTER the lapse of more than a year, Miss Wight resumes her journal, and continues it at intervals until near the close of 1849.

" *Oct. 12, 1848.* While Mrs. F. was sitting with us this evening Laura said to her, ' Your voice sounds like a man's.' On being asked her reasons for thinking so, she replied that she *saw*, putting her hand on her throat. The lady has a deep voice."

Speaking of her health, Miss Wight says : —

" She has a good appetite and is in excellent spirits, or as she told me to-day, ' I have a hundred good spirits, but you have only ten.'

" *Nov. 4.* In giving her a lesson to-day upon the origin of laws and government, and the penalties attached by men to the breaking of these laws, she asked with great earnestness, ' Why did our Father make men to do wrong and to suffer so much?'

" She says much lately of being independent and earning her own living when she leaves school, but the thought of going home to live seems to have no place in her plans for the future. She grows continually more affectionate, more lovely, and at the same time more sensitive.

" *Nov. 10.* I had a very pleasant conversation with Laura this morning. She told me of her prayers ; how calm and happy it made her to pray. Her prayer, as she repeated it to me, was beautiful from its simplicity and fitness. I wish I could recall her words, for the form of expression was very perfect, but I could not ask her to repeat it. She asked, ' Can you realize that God is with us and takes care of us constantly ? ' She spoke of death : ' I cannot imagine how my spirit can feel without my body. I do not know why I should not feel willing to die, but I do not feel willing.' But notwithstanding all these misgivings which arise in her mind occasionally as she thinks of the future, she feels that existence is a great blessing. She said, as often before, ' I am so glad that I was created ! ' Indeed, when in health there is not a happier being in existence than she. She asked, ' Can we conceive how great and good God is ? ' ' How industrious he is ! ' she exclaimed when we had been talking of his goodness as manifested in the creation of all things around us. ' Did you know that my heart has much more love for everybody than last year? I am very much happier. When I meet people and they kiss me so hard, they are so very kind to me and I laugh and feel so much more kind and loving.' "

Under another date she says : —

" Laura has become much interested in Free Soil principles, and few voters have made more earnest inquiries into the character of the candidates for the Presidency. It was with difficulty that I convinced her that a man might have some good qualities even though he were a slave-holder and were willing to fight, and indeed, I doubt whether I did really succeed She asked why her father should not be a slave as well as the negroes. She could see no reason why one man who worked hard should not be a slave as well as another.

"*Nov. 16.* She made a remark that made me realize, more then ever, her privations. 'I want to do right, but I cannot hear with my ears what everybody says about it; what they think is right and best to do.' She said this more seriously than she usually speaks of her own peculiarities.

"Reading in Laura's journal that her heart was almost broken by the loss of a dear friend who had gone away. I asked her if I should get some glue to mend it. With a half-serious, half-comic expression she replied, ' Time will be the best glue.'

"*Jan. 29, 1849.* This morning I read one of Dr. Peabody's sermons to Laura, ' We know but in part.' She was much pleased that she could understand it so readily. She clasped the book with delight, and said, ' I wish it was mine, for it would always fill my heart with love and goodness. I am so glad that Dr. (Howe) took so much trouble to find out how to teach me to give me the best education. If I had studied all the time I should have made more progress. Why did you not teach me when I was poor (thin) and had a cough?'

"*April 10.* She said to-day, ' How glad I am that our minds are made to go thousands of miles to see our friends and be with them, though they are so remote.' (She had just parted with a friend to whom she was much attached and who was going to reside in

California.) A few moments after she asked, 'Will
our minds all be alike, when they go to heaven away
from our bodies? I think they will be exactly alike.
How hard it is to think God has lived forever! If
we were all alike we could not know each other. I
think we shall know our friends and much better than
we do here, but I have not naturally much confidence
in God. Christ had the most confidence in God, he
was willing to be killed. Do you think he feels like
himself now in heaven? Do we think as much of our
only Father as we ought to? Does it not give you
more love in your heart to think much of him? It
does me.'

"For a few weeks past I have been often struck
with her apparent appreciation of unexpressed thoughts.
Anything that interests me deeply seems to suggest a
corresponding train of thought in her. It is so often
the case that I can scarcely believe it to be the effect
of accident merely. Her parting advice to her friend,
Mrs. F., was, 'I hope you will be very happy & useful & loving & kind always; & also that you will
have reverence & respect for all human beings. I
feel in my heart that you will strive to do your duty to
God, & it will please him so much to see you doing
the most good to all in the world. I shall wish to hear
of your happiness, & of the country, etc., so much.
You must think of me & ask for my sympathy &
confidence when you are troubled and homesick in
mind & heart. You must not think I shall forget
you in my life if I do not write to you frequently.'

"*April 26.* She attended a wedding for the first
time. She conducted herself with the most perfect pro-

priety and expressed her good wishes very gracefully, giving as well as receiving much pleasure.

" This afternoon she alluded to the incident in her early childhood of throwing the cat into the fire. I asked her if she knew she was doing wrong at the time. She said, ' Not till my mother punished me, then I knew it was wrong.' "

In August she spent some weeks with her dear friends in Billerica, and while there, wrote a long letter to her brother Addison to whom she was much attached. She sympathized with him in his love of study, and indulged in dreams of a future time coming when she would be able to study with him. She appreciated her superiority in age, and occasionally assumed the position of adviser. She had just heard that he enjoyed using a gun sometimes.

The following is a copy of the letter:—

BILLERICA. Aug. 26, 1849.

MY DEAREST BROTHER ADDISON:

I wish you a very happy Sunday. I came to Billerica last Friday, P. M. I was highly delighted to get a kind note from you. My little heart was filled with numerous delightful emotions. I did not approve of our killing the most huge bird. But he was so intensely cruel as to kill those poultry which existed very happily. If I were you I would hate to hurt any living thing, because my heavenly father is so infinitely kind & benevolent as to have all things in order. I am very grateful to him, for he presented my brothers

& sisters & numerous great blessings. God is always very much displeased to see any one hurt birds,
or anything that lives very happily. I am positively
sure that it is very wrong for you & John to like to
hurt or kill the happy creatures. I am extremely sad
that you love such cruel fun so dearly in that way. I
am very sure you would be much happier during your
existence if you will only not be selfish & cruel to
hurt or do any wrong thing in the world. I am very
kind & amiable in my own heart. I wish to give you
some very good instruction with all my heart. I love
goodness very much. I wish you would strive to
resist such temptations in hunting & hurting. Will
you exert yourself to regard my great wishes? I do
not doubt in the least it will increase your happiness if
you would cultivate your benevolence and patience very
resolutely. You must learn to control your bad habits
entirely. It will strengthen your mind greatly. Did
you ever feel unkind or unamiable towards me in your
heart while you staid with me? I never allow myself
to be vexed or impatient or unamiable. I hope you will
always have much love and sympathy for your dear
eldest sister & all human beings. I do not really
censure you, but I wish to give you very good influence
or instruction. I hope that you will be so very grateful to me for my advice.

God is so infinitely good who sends us a very immense number of beautiful flowers, etc. I had very
many roses, etc., this summer. They were so very
sweet & elegant, that my desire was very great to
fly & exhibit them to you all. I considered that
you would admire them very much. I love beau-

ties very dearly. I do not think you love beauties & goodness. I am very sad more frequently this year than I used to be. It is hard to explain the causes or cases. My mind seems rather weak and sad. I like sympathy very much in sorrow and joys. Did you have much confidence in me that I would fulfil my promise of writing you a letter? I knit you a chain with great pleasure last month, & hope you will like it. Will you please to wear it to remember me very kindly? I recite seven or eight lessons to Miss Wight regularly. Wight reads to me in the Bible for a while. Then she reads to me from my precious book, the title is " The King's Messengers." I have an hour to study till breakfast; at quarter of seven. I study Algebra. Geometry, Physiology, N. Philosophy, History. Last month I implored Wight to please to teach me Algebra & Geometry. She said that it was very difficult for me to study them. G. seems very difficult for me to comprehend it perfectly. I have a great deal of perseverance & patience. I love to study G. & A. with very great zeal & alacrity continually. When I first studied G., Wight was very kind & patient to explain to me the meaning of all of those things so repeatedly for a week. I thought that it was impossible to understand G., but I rejoice very much to be able to puzzle out at last. You & I love studies so very much. I should love to come & study with you much, alone sometimes. I fear that you would drive me out of your presence. For I think you did not like to sit & commune with me in the least. You used to avoid me many times when I wished to be with you with my heart. All of my friends are very sociable & affectionate to me. It gives

me great pleasure to see them around me. I think you
like to receive letters from me better than to see or talk
with me. . . . I shall delight much to have a long
& full letter from you as soon as you are at leisure to
reply to my letter. I send my very best love to you.
Do write to me spry. I wish you a very sweet &
happy eve.

L. D. BRIDGMAN.

If any one avoid her or dislike to talk with her,
she notices it very quickly, but in this respect her
brothers, when young, were not unlike most
children, who instinctively shrink from any one
whom they perceive to have a natural defect or to
be peculiar in any way, and she was at home with
them so little they did not have time to overcome
this feeling.

In September we find her resuming her studies.

"*Sept. 17.* Speaking of the importation of tea, coffee,
and spices, she asked, Do you think they are important?' 'Not to me, I do not like to use them.' Looking,
very thoughtful she said, 'But they were made: why
were they created if they were not meant to be used?'
At another time she inquired why her mother was not
so fond of adorning her house as I was, and said, ' I am
more fond of beauties than of anything else in the world.'
'Except goodness,' I suggested. With a smile she
said, ' I meant goodness was the greatest beauty of all.'

"*Sept. 18.* She asked, ' Do you think we shall be
homesick when we leave this earth as we are when we
leave our homes?'

"*Sept. 19.* She was very quick in algebra this morn-ing. There is a great difference in her at different times, and without any apparent reason. One morning the most trifling thing will be a stumbling-block in her way, and the very next day she will seem to grasp a diffi-culty of the same nature with ease.

"*Nov. 1.* Her arithmetic lesson was not very good. From the beginning she has disliked this study. I told her that everything which gives the mind strength, even the study of arithmetic, increases our power to appre-ciate goodness, and will make our lives more useful and happy. To remind her of Jesus seldom fails to bring her into a right frame of mind. After this conversa-tion, I gave her another question, which she solved suc-cessfully. She asked why she was not naturally as good as other people. I told her we all had faults, and that I could see in her many good qualities. She re-plied, ' But you do not know how unamiable I am, for often when I try to smile, and you think I am amiable, I have impatient feelings in my heart.' Later in the day we talked of the difference between reason and in-stinct. I told her that reason could see the connection between cause and effect which instinct could not. She reminded me of the story of the elephant, who, on being pricked by a tailor, filled his trunk with water which he discharged upon the tailor. This seemed to her to show reason.

"*Nov. 6.* She was very successful in arithmetic, and I asked how it was she was so bright. She said, ' I think an angel came from heaven and made my mind more bright.'

"*Nov. 8.* Laura is certainly improving. She has

surprised me all day by her quickness of apprehension
and power of application. She has waked up, though
it can hardly be said of such a mind as hers that it is
ever asleep; but to-day, as I was talking to her about
active and passive states of mind, she laughed, and said
she could understand the difference very easily, for she
knew it by experience.

" *Nov. 10.* Finished the reading of Jarvis's Physiology, and now lay it aside for a few months, as I have
found best to do with other books. After an interval
of time she seems to look at the subjects in a new light,
and things once difficult become easy to her."

With these extracts we close the journal of
Miss Wight.

We add one more leaf from Laura's journal of
December, in which she tells of her plans for a
Christmas party : —

" I have had many very pleasant and comical thoughts
to-day. I anticipate having (an) extremely pleasant
festival time on Christmas. I should be most delighted
to celebrate the day. I would send a very cordial invitation to my dear family. I should wish Miss Wight
to assist me to write many notes, for the purpose of
inviting them, two days before. I can bear such exhil-
aration with all my heart and mind. I must purchase
a very big and elegant Christmas tree. I should be
very much absorbed in business. I could suspend
fruits & very tiny baskets containing sweetmeats on the
branches of the trees. I shall wish to promote the happiness of my visitors as much as I could. I think that if

one hundred of my friends assembled to our new spacious parlor, the room would be so very full indeed. & the air would be scanty or breathed up totally. I could have a very big table & have it set very richly. I could have all kinds of pies, & cake, & fruit on the table. Afterward I should like to make my visitors laugh very heartily by my most comical remarks. I could ask Mr. P. to loan me his musical box, that my friends may have the pleasure of hearing very sweet & loud & soft sounds, as long as they liked We shall sit up till eleven or twelve in the eve. How can I assign a plenty of beds to them? 1 shall be impelled (compelled) to deposit some bed clothes on the floors for them to repose themselves upon. One of them might be compelled to immerse into my little bathing closet. She will be very much exhausted from standing so long a time. She will be apt to nod her head all night. She would not find herself half so much refreshed in the morning, as if she had slept in bed. Some of the friends will have to sleep on my shelves. I should be very sad to compel them to sleep so uncomfortably and uneasily. I am enjoying this castle in the air very much. I am naturally very fond of mirthfulness."

In the above extract she alludes to a music box. She sometimes had this box loaned to her and took much pleasure in placing it in a chair, and then putting her feet upon the rounds of the chair so that she ' could feel it play.'

Miss Wight continued to teach Laura until the spring of 1850. Five years of uninterrupted teaching, of a kind which drew most heavily upon the nervous system, had so prostrated her that she was obliged to resign her charge. That it was a sad trial to both teacher and pupil need not be told after the preceding record.

Some months later Laura was obliged to bid her a long farewell as she sailed for a new home in the Sandwich Islands, and to relinquish also the bright hopes she had so long cherished of helping her take care of "some nice little house," and living always with her.

In Dr. Howe's Eighteenth Report, made January, 1850, he speaks of the position which Laura held before the world at this time, as follows : —

" Her progress has been a curious and an interesting spectacle. She has come into human society with a sort of triumphal march; her course has been a perpetual ovation. Thousands have been watching her with eager eyes, and applauding each successful step, while she, all unconscious of their gaze, holding on to the slender thread, and feeling her way along, has advanced with faith and courage towards those who awaited her with trembling hope. Nothing shows more than her case the importance which, despite their useless waste of human life and human capacity, men really attach to a human soul. They owe to her something for furnishing an opportunity of showing how much of goodness there is in them ; for surely the way in which she has been regarded is creditable to humanity. Perhaps there are not three living women whose names are more widely known than hers ; and there is not one who has excited so much sympathy and interest. There are thousands of women in the world who are striving to attract its notice and gain its admiration, some by the natural magic of beauty and grace, some by high nobility of talent, some by the lower nobility of rank and title, some by the vulgar show of wealth ; but none of them has done it so effectually as this poor blind, deaf, and dumb girl, by the silent show of her misfortunes, and her successful efforts to surmount them.

" The treatment she has received shows something of human progress too ; for the time was, when a child, bereaved of senses as she is, would have been regarded as a monster and treated as a burden and a curse, even among the most civilized people of the world; she would, perhaps, have been thrown into the river, or exposed upon the mountain to wild beasts. But now there are millions of people by whom it is recognized as a duty and esteemed as a privilege to protect and cherish her, or any one in like situation.

" There is something, perhaps, in the rarity of such cases of manifold bereavement, something in the fact that she is the first person who ever came out of such a dark and silent prison to tell us plainly of its condition, something of pride in the proof which she gives in the native power of the human soul ; but still, bating all this, the amount of tender sympathy in her misfortunes and of real interest in the attempt to lighten them which has been shown by thousands of sensitve hearts is most gratifying to reflect upon."

CHAPTER XVIII.

WE depart from our chronological order to re-late some items of interest occurring during the last few years which have not been reported in the journals. We shall be able to give only a frag-mentary history of her subsequent life, no further record having been kept.

In the summer of 1846, after an absence of a year, I returned to Boston to reside, and Laura was made happy by having another place to visit. Nothing ever gave her more pleasure than to be left alone and allowed to examine things at leis-ure; and having once been led through my house, she required no further assistance in her explora-tions, but was soon familiar not only with the rooms, but with closets and bureaus. Her great gentleness and delicacy of touch made it entirely safe to trust her with the most valued treasures, and I never knew her to injure anything.

One day she proved to me that she knew more about my possessions than I did myself. She asked me to give her a piece of silk for some pur-pose, and when told I had only a few pieces that were like my dresses, and could not spare them, said, "You are mistaken, in the closet in the third story there is a box, and it has in it some pieces that are not like your dresses." I sent her to find them, and to my surprise she was right. Nothing could be misplaced in the house without her perceiving it.

She was always pleased with children and liked to hold an infant in her arms, and her joy was great when she was told there was a baby in our house. She watched its growth and development with the greatest interest, and was very happy to bring a present of the tiniest shoes to be found. In her journal of Jan. 23, she writes of baby's first visit to her: "I was very pleasantly detained by visitors. Mrs. L. and little Mary came to spend the P. M. with us. I was so highly delighted to have such pleasant company. I derived so much pleasure from giving so constant attention to my cunning pet. I led her about the work room and our room. I loved to carry the child in my arms about very much. I willingly let her hear my musical box play for a while. When I took it away from her it caused her to cry instantly, because she disliked to give the music up. We went to the shop to put the child on the scales and to let the blind boys see her. I was very sorry to have her go home."

After hearing of the death of little Mary, she wrote in her journal: "I had a great many sad thoughts in my mind to-day, my dear friend's only little daughter has died. I used to love & caress her when she was a very little babe very much, as if she was my own child. I used to call her my little pet, etc." She wrote the following letter without suggestion from any one : —

SEPT. 28, 1849.

MY DEAR MRS. L.:

I was very much surprised to hear of the decease of your darling last Tuesday. I hoped she would recover very soon. I trust that your little Mary is much happier at her new home than she was on earth. I am very positive God and His beloved Son, Christ, will educate your child much better than men could in this world. I can scarcely realize that the school is so excessively beautiful in heaven. I can sympathize with you in your great affliction. I cannot help thinking of your trouble and little Mary's illness. I know very certainly that God will promote her happiness forever. I loved her very dearly, as if she were my own daughter. I shall miss her very much every time I come to see you. I send my best love to you and a kiss. I am very sad for you.

Yours,   L. B.

After Miss Wight left, she had no regular lessons. Some of the blind girls were asked to talk with her at certain hours, but, with the oversight of the matron, she was left to occupy her time as she liked. She had reached the age of twenty-one, and her intellectual development was such that it was not considered necessary she should have a person entirely devoted to her. At one time the experiment was tried of employing a young person about her own age as companion, but without satisfactory result; she preferred to be alone. The books in raised type were her companions, and the Bible was her special delight. She found more time now to devote to her work, and as there was always a ready sale for everything she could make, she was stimulated to do even more than was best for her health. She enjoyed visiting her old teachers and a few other friends, with whom she carried on a regular correspondence.

She sympathized warmly with her friends in affliction, and her letters written on such occasions are very touching. Some of these are kindly loaned me for publication. The extracts are copied as they came from her pencil, save that the punctuation is somewhat changed to make the sense more apparent.

SUNNY HOME, Jan. 25th, 1853.

MY DEAR SISTER, MISS ROGERS:

I received your most kind letter last Thursday, with the greatest of pleasure. . . . I was so sadly & violently surprised to hear of (the death of) your lovely sister Mary, last Nov., the same day of my arrival from my dear home. I sympathize with you very truly in your greatest afflictions. I wish very much to console you. I rejoice so greatly for your

22

heart's sake that Harriet is with you. She is in E's place now. She will be your own constant companion, I hope. She will be of such a great comfort to you as the sun (that) shines. I did not dream that you would be attacked by an other loss so suddenly. (Alluding to the death of a little sister previously.) I know of course that your darling Mary is much happier in seeing her own little Ella, at a new home which belongs to God. M. loves you so much more than while she dwelt on this big world. Mary watches you much more, & knows how you feel in her loss. She will however smile upon you like an Angel.

God will educate her with much more love & beauty & meekness, than these men (could do) who are most religious & benevolent on the earth.

Christ will treat M & E so very justly & with greatest refinement, & also will have such a beautiful influence upon them both forever. M. is very truly happy to live with Ella & other friends You will always miss Mary very sorrowfully, but I delight so highly in the thought of her being delivered from her sufferings, by God, who was absolutely merciful & lovely. Mary used to smile upon you very sweetly always. I love her excessively, as if she were my own Sister. I cannot believe of the idea that you wish Mary to return back for your own comfort & pleasure. . . .

It was her habit, after she was without a teacher, to keep in her mind long lists of words, and bring them to me for explanation. On the occasion of her visits she was jealous of every interruption, whether from children or visitors, and often recommended that the former should remain in the nursery, and the latter be told I was engaged. She could not afford to lose a moment from conversation. Those who were now about her at the Institution had had comparatively little experience in talking with the fingers; she was always patient with the slowest talker, yet it was a pleasure to her that she could make her fingers fly once more, and be understood. She liked to consult me about her clothing, and in brief to come as a daughter to a mother. On one occasion I had led her to her chamber and bade her good night. Hearing her moving about for an hour after, I went to see what she was doing. On opening the door cautiously I saw that bed, chairs, and table were covered with the articles of a wedding *trousseau* which she had found in the bureau drawers. I said to her, " It is eleven o'clock. Why have you so many clothes about?" She replied, "I was going to ask you to-morrow to go with me and buy a great many yards of cotton, and I want you to cut it into many things. I do not like the patterns I have, and I knew your nice things were in these drawers, so I have been trying them all on; those that I like are on the table, and I will put the others away." It was with difficulty that I ;ould answer her as seriously as she felt the occasion required, but I promised to do as she wished the next day if she would go quickly to bed.

On another occasion a clergyman arrived unexpectedly as we were leaving the tea-table. I left Laura abruptly, to prepare a cup of tea for him before he went to perform a wedding service, for which he had travelled some distance. When I returned to her, I explained to her the cause of my absence, saying, "Prof. P. has gone to marry a couple." She was standing, and at once raised herself on her toes, and with a look of the greatest disgust on her face, thrust out her arm to its full length, and spelled with her fingers "f-o-o-l." For an instant I was puzzled to find a reason for such severe condemnation and unusual display of feeling, but on thinking of my sentence, I perceived that while I had made use of a common expression, it was one with which, perhaps, she had never met before, and therefore had understood me that he had come to Boston to be married himself, and to a couple of wives. It was not strange that her sense of propriety should be outraged.

In the summer of 1852 she returned to her father's house in Hanover with the understanding that this was to be her permanent home. She had always enjoyed her visits there, but now, when 'he novelty had worn off, she became very lonely, and missed sadly her old surroundings. In the large family in which the greater part of her life had been passed, there was always some one with whom she could have a social chat. She was interested in everybody, and to an incredible extent knew what was passing about her. The transition to the quiet life of a small family was more than her sensitive nature could bear. In the winter following she lost all inclination for food, but complained of nothing, and probably did not know the cause of her increasing debility. At last she was confined to her bed, and Dr. Howe was notified of her condition. He found her almost at death's door, but with no disease save homesickness. He sent a lady to bring her back to the Institution, which was accomplished with difficulty, and as she was carried into her old room, and laid upon her bed, she looked as though her spirit had already fled. She began to improve immediately, but required much care for a long time. For many years she continued to occupy the same room, and was a happy member of the family. She went into the school-room at certain hours, when she could share the instruction in writing, etc., given to the blind girls.

She has always manifested strong likes and dislikes. A pleasing young girl of sixteen, who had become temporarily blind, was carried to the Institution. Laura conceived a violent affection for her which developed singularly. She appointed herself both guardian and nurse, and refused to allow any one else to do anything for her, showing much jealousy if it was attempted. At last, to make sure of no interruption, she locked herself into the room with her, and for many hours no one could gain admittance. She is especially attracted to those who have a gentle, timid nature, which she discovers at once. Her ability to read character is very remarkable, and she is rarely mistaken. When it is remembered that this is done at the fingers' ends, it would not be strange if this statement were received with incredulity, but every one who has known her intimately will attest its truth. As has been said, " She observes the *tones* of the finger language," and these are as pronounced to her as those of the voice are to our ears. She knows how different people laugh, and often speaks of the sweet smile of one and another. It may be thought that she must be always feeling of the face, and thus make herself disagreeable; but this is not so, she rarely touches it, and yet judges correctly. There was at one time in the house a very gentlemanly young man who was not blind. He was well dressed, and his appearance did not betray the deficiency of intellect which really existed. Laura had not met him until the day he was introduced to her. He could not speak with his fingers, so it was merely a shaking of hands that passed between them. Instantly after she dropped his hand she raised hers, letting the fingers hang down, and said to the person who introduced her, " Is he a fool? "

One day she called to see a friend to whom she was attached and met her husband for the first time. He was a man highly esteemed, but very reserved and distant in manner. She shook hands with him and asked, " Has he many friends? Is he greatly beloved in his own family? Is he severe? "

It was a cause of surprise to those who were constantly with her that it so often happened that while sitting quietly at work, apparently absorbed by her own thoughts, she should ask some question directly bearing upon the subject of general conversation, to which no one had given her any clew. This led to the remark, " Laura always knows our thoughts."

She takes notice of dress, and likes to examine it sufficiently to get an idea of the pattern, but shows her good taste by choosing for herself both material and style which are appropriate. She had desired to have a silk dress, and was much pleased on receiving one from a friend on her return from Europe, its value being enhanced from the fact that she could speak of it as her " dress from Paris." This was not because Paris is the headquarters of fashion, but because there was, to her mind, something akin to romance pertaining to everything she had learned in geography. She had wished also for a watch. This may seem to be a superfluity for a deaf and dumb and blind person, but she easi'y learned to tell the time, and enjoyed using one which was loaned to her, always placing it under her pillow at night, and claiming that it waked her at the right time in the morning. A few years since, through the generosity of a couple of friends, she was presented with a watch in a hunter's case, the crystal being removed that she might have more ready access to the hands. She has derived much enjoyment as well as companionship from it.

From the fact of her having been the recipient of such special care and attention during all her life, we should hardly think her blameworthy if she should be thoughtless of others and careful to guard her own interests; but on the contrary, she has an affectionate disposition, and nothing has delighted her more throughout her life than to be able to assist a friend or to send some comfort to a poor person. At the time of the famine in Ireland her sympathies were much moved, and she purchased, with the proceeds of her own industry, a barrel of flour, which was sent to the sufferers.

About the year 1855 it was suggested to Laura that she write an account of events which she could remember in her life at home, before she came to the Institution. We copy extracts from this paper, trusting that the quaintness of her style will give interest even to a twice-told tale :—

"I shall like very much indeed to write the life of my childhood. I can remember of a great many circum-

stances & events which occurred in my earliest days.
I was born in Hanover, N. H., the 21st of Dec. 1829.
I had one brother named Milo, & two first sisters
Mary & Frances Collina. They all left my lovely home,
& went to a spiritual land to live with my heavenly
Father. I never knew them except what I have heard
about since then. Mary & Frances were attacked by
the perilous fever scarlet, which was a cause of their
death. Little Milo was born with the nature of great
weakness; he was carried from his dear mother's sight
in the arms of an angel, when three months old.
. . . I was two years & a few months old when I
was in the calamity of a raging fever, which was scarlet, I was very sorely ill for three long weeks. . . .
I could not take a morsel of bread or cracker, neither
could swallow throughin my little throat for a few long
weeks, except that I drank some very nourishing liquid,
crust coffee. I was not conveyed in one's arms out of
doors, even for an instant, for three or four months. I
recollect very distinctly how much I used to lay (lie)
in a nice old cradle on account of the illness & weakness. I liked to have some one rock me along in it
extremely continually. . . . One day I was repos-
ing my little body in that snug cradle, a spark of coals
with fire flew very lightly upon my neck, & the flame
of fire spread to my chin (so) that it rendered (made)
both of my neck & chin grow closely, but the inflamma-
tion went off, & it caused a scar on the skin. My dear
mother kept watching over me in another person's
lap on the occasion of suffering. I kept sobbing very
hard unconsciously. I took some sugar saturated with
some peppermint, I liked very much, for a sort of

medicine. . . . I was born in fragile health. I
was very fond of all sorts of tricks in my childhood.
I had a good deal of distress with my eyes for months,
they would not bear the rays of light an instant, from
which I tried to prevent. I put up my hands over my
ill eyes, & rush(ed) into a very snug bedroom for a
bit of darkness. The nerve was painful that effectually
made a great shower of tears in my eyes, which finally
gushed out at once. It was from ignorance of the fact,
that I imagined, that the sun always shone beneath,
through the floor in my mother's kitchen upon which I
reflect with my eye, near her right window. I was
perfectly unwise, & very unfortunate about the wisdom
of God & his beloved Son Jesus. I did not have such
a doll at the earliest period of my childhood. My
mother knew nothing about dolls for many long years.
I never had play-toys for amusements, or a pleasure
except what I contrived to find in her house for myself
to play. I had many pleasant times in sporting. I
could not articulate, or see, or hear. (Afterwards) I
had a very funny doll made of a lot of rags, which
pleased me very much indeed, that homely doll was
bound very nicely & smoothly. I had some neat
clothes for the doll to dress in. I never gave the doll
a name, for I did not know of the fact that such dolls
could receive any name, & also, I was not educated
how to use my little fingers. My mother was not
capable of learning the finger alphabet for numerous long years. We never had a dream of the invention for a way to spell a shortest or easiest word with
the fingers in the world. I used to make some signs
for my mother, what I wished her to know of, it was

not a least shadow between her and I, as she could comprehend all signs I made. . . . . I had a small thin plate for my own, it was a gift from an old man named Mr. Asa Tenny whom I always loved & respected so greatly, my first and old benefactor. The nice tin plate has the finger alphabet printed in raised letters around on the edge. I occupied my plate at the table frequently. I could not have practised in reading the blind (raised) letters with my fingers for various reasons, until I was brought up to an education, when I was almost eight years old. . . Mr. Tenny was always very patient and kind and gentle to me. He used to stroke my face with his finger for caress, & also let me know him. He had a most original manner of taking hold of my arms before I could have touched his hands & recognized him. As I felt his hat upon his head, I knew him instantly always. The hat was very common, so plain & sleek & durable, it seems to have felt to my fingers like a piece of paste board. Mr. T. always dressed in most simple & refugal (frugal) clothes. I had two little chairs, one of those chairs had rockers & they both had arms. I sat in them a good deal which I enjoyed exceedingly. . . . I derived a great pleasure from walking & rambling & sporting with Mr. T. daily. He used to go with me out of the doors in search of eggs very frequently. I liked so much to grope in hollowed nests with my little hands, seeking for a single egg. Mr. T. commanded me not to rob the poor hen of her very last egg, by a gesture which I understood so clearly, but I did not know the reason why he left one egg remaining undisturbed in the position. He influenced me with something like geography, which was, that I flinged sand, stones & gravels & branches of aged trees into the brook. I enjoyed that game extremely. He would conduct me to call on his friends as often as was his convenience, or my mother approved of my going with him. He was my first benefactor on this earth. He was stout & firm to lift me up in his big arms a long distance from place to place. I admired very much to be carried in his arms like a babe. We went out to pluck lots of different berries at any rate (to any amount?) that we pleased. I was always disposed to subsist on them, mixed with most luxurious milk & white or brown-bread or crackers. Mr. T. never liked to scold me for doing a little thing which was really wrong according to his opinion. He never inflict(ed) **a punishment upon me in his life.**"

CHAPTER XIX.

In 185 she made the acquaintance of Katie Hill, a blind girl who had just arrived from Germany, and had become a member of the school. She was especially attracted to her because, in her early years, she had been much attached to the wife and children of our German music-teacher. They had returned to the Fatherland, and this girl was at once received with affection for their sake.

At this time Laura was in the habit of convers ing with the blind girls freely, and very soon taught her the finger alphabet. Katie had had little opportunity for acquiring knowledge of books, not having been at any school for the blind, but she had learned to love the Saviour, and "had done," as she expressed it, "some missionary work." In conversing with Laura it was very natural to her to talk of Christ, and the ideas which she gave her were different from any she had previously received. In her visits to me she talked much about her " new sister Katie," and told me of what she was learning from her. She wrote a very interesting letter to her old friend Mrs. H. in

Germany, telling her how much she loved her new German friend and of what she had taught her. Unfortunately this letter, which she brought to me to forward, was not copied, and the original has not been preserved, but several persons to whom it was read by me, remember it distinctly as a very remarkable letter.

In her occasional visits to me she always spoke freely of her interest in reading the Bible, but the great Teacher led her to an appropriation of its truths through deep sorrow.

In 1860 she heard of the sudden death of her eldest sister. I did not see her at this time, and know of her experience only through others. There seems to have arisen first a spirit of rebellion against God, and she continued for months to cherish bitter feelings, and to shun conversation on religious topics, which had previously been her delight. Just how long this state of mind lasted we have no knowledge, but the following letter shows the conflict ended, and an entire change of feeling : —

Sunny Home, Mar. 10, 61.

My very dear Miss Rogers :

I am so happy to devote a little time to write you a letter this lovely day. Behold what manner of glory & love & grace our holy God hath bestowed upon us. We can appreciate his kindness. Let us thank him for whatsoever he gives us with all our hearts. May the

Lord be with you forever & ever. Grace be with you. Amen.

This is a prayer for my true friend from me. I am better this morn. I have not been well much of the time this Winter & in the Fall But I am much happier in mind concerning God & his begotten Son, Jesus Christ. I profess religion since last spring most fervently. I devote a great deal of my time to studying the sacred Bible. I rejoice so highly that God has helped me how to comprehend his works in many ways. I can not comprehend some of his works, but a part of his gracious work. I read in the blessed Bible daily, which I prize the most of all books in this world. My spirit is much stronger than my bodily strength. . . . I wish much to meet you once more. I would be so joyful to pass many long weeks with you. Please to let me know about your leisure for a visit from your old pupil L. B.

I am in such raptures on account of my chosen friend Wight, who is expected home in July with her family. Miss M. saw Mr. Wight in town last week; he proposed to her that I should go to Wayland & visit Mrs. Bond as soon as she recruited her rest. He longs for her. Yours truly.

L. Bridgman.

Her old teacher, Miss Wight (Mrs. Bond), returned from the Sandwich Islands with her family in 1861, after an absence of five years. Laura was not told of her arrival, but was summoned from the dinner-table to see a friend. She shook hands with her, not recognizing her for an instant, but the next moment she sprang from the floor in her delight, and fell nearly fainting into her arms.

During a visit to Hanover in the summer of 1863, she was baptized and received to membership in the Baptist Church, with which her parents were connected.   Later in the year, while visiting her friends in Billerica, she talked much about her recent baptism, and was asked to write an account of it.   She complied with this request, prefacing it with an account of her feelings on the death of her sister.

JAN. 8, 1864.

MY VERY DEAR FRIEND:

I am most happy to have the utmost pleasure to write you a sketch concerning myself.

One Sabbath day of February 4th long years ago (1860), I heard from my old homestead by the interpretation of my dear friend, Miss Moulton.   She received a letter concerning my oldest sister Mary from my dear mother.   As Miss Moulton had reported a fate of death of my precious sister Mary, I burst into a bad cry, my heart ached so painfully; it was broken with a great crush.   Many tears rushed with a heavy shower from my eyes.   I could hardly spell a word with my fingers for many hours.   My soul was cumbered and cast down.   In spirit I was unable to bear such vast afflictions, it was the great torment of my heart, which caused me a great trial, to suffer the loss of my dear sister Mary.   Miss Moulton was so kind & attentive to me in such distressing pain & sorrow in spirit.   She took me with all her strength from her sitting room up to my cozy room. It was hard for me to guide myself alone, for I trembled of great agitation and pain, but the Lord was good & merciful, & a firm staff to my comfort. He was my gracious and holy guide. I was not a Christian at that time. Miss Moulton put me on my cozy bed, and did so much for my comfort. She wiped the tears from my face, though they ran so freely from my eyes. . . . I had a very sorrowful Sunday, contemplating the prospect of death of my dear sister Mary all the day long. I was indisposed to relish my meals, on account of the idea of my suffering sorrow & affliction for weeks. It seems as if there could never be peace or happiness in the vast world, that I might obtain to my soul for a great while. I did not feel reconciliation to my Heavenly Father or his blest son Jesus, whose grace, & mercy, & love (was shown) in calling Mary forth unto a land of bliss & glory, I loved my sister so dearly. I could not trust in God and Jesus, as much as I do now. I dwelt in a condition of unhappiness & despair, many weeks. My head was laid upon a pillow of grief and lamentation many nights. My slumber was brittle and frail, as my head was heavy laden with various notions concerning my loved Mary. I wrote a letter to my poor mother consoling her in her anguish, etc. While I wrote it my tears gently rolled from my eyes, & my heart ached sadly. Miss Moulton came to comfort my broken heart, by repeating some verses of the fourteenth chapter of John, one Sabbath in April, after the death of Mary. I began to review a (the) subject of my Saviour Jesus & baptism. I did not feel inclined to ask my mamma any questions concerning baptism. I only asked mother, how a person was bap-

23

tized with water. In May, it came to pass that I thought more and more of my Redeemer & baptism. I abode with my mother a month in a new house, and then I departed from my poor mother. My dear brother John escorted me to Thetford, Vt. I staid with my dear cousin Emily for more than three months. I attained much enjoyment of conversing with my cousin about such sacred things. I thought how delightful it might have been to my soul if I could be baptized in the pure water by the minister who usually preached the Holy Ghost to the blest church in Thetford, Vt. But my dear God did not approve of my doing that away from my home. I felt fearful at times from these thoughts concerning the performance of baptism I thought that there was danger of sinking my head beneath the water, & I might be drowned in the depth of water. I did not feel strong and confident sufficiently for being in a grave. In June three years ago (1860), on my abode with cousin Emily I was permitted to meet a certain woman by the loving kindness of my Saviour. My heart promptly received her in the holy name of my Saviour Jesus Christ, who opened my heart, & illumined it with his light. He put his nature upon me so that I should leave all evil things, & love good things by the spirit of the grace of Jesus our Saviour. I felt so cold & impure in heart, I wished to run away from my cousin, one day when the woman was present with her. My cousin claimed (wished) me to remain with her on purpose to get acquainted with that beloved woman. By mercy & love of God, he ordained that pious lady & I to be true friends. She is my blessed and adopted grandmother now. In the fall I had much delight in a religious conversation with my dear adopted sister, & her husband, & my dear mother. One sunny P. M. in July two years ago, I visited my adopted sister Mrs. H. We had a very solemn happiness with a talk in the library with Mr. H., a most excellent minister. We transacted some business concerning the sacred ordinance. My sister Mrs. Herrick called upon me the first Saturday of July (1863), she interpreted some sentiments to me for the reverend. Shortly after dinner I accompanied my mother to his house a few rods from my home. I had a happy call there, till it was time for us all to go to the holy sanctuary, to attribute prayers & holy communion to the Almighty Father. The holy church agreed to vote me a member. The 6th of July, the first Sabbath, my cousin Mary called to see me once or twice Sunday. I went with her & my mother to Mr. Herrick's house at noon. I was so glad to meet a few ladies there, I was waited upon by those ladies in preparation for baptism. I could hardly help myself undress, & dress myself. Mr. H. welcomed me so gladly at his house. I was guided to the brookside by my mamma & Mrs. Huntington. Mr. H. sent for me one of his chairs to sit by the side of the brook, while holy prayer was being addressed. Two students sang a hymn 112. I believe that the first line of the hymn is

" In all my God's appointed ways."

I did not feel inclined to talk with my fingers at the blessed ordinance, but I was so happy to have my mother or any person speak to me. My soul was overwhelmed with spiritual joy and light in the presence of God and his blest son Jesus Christ. I could hardly smile, for I felt solemnly happy. I could reflect (upon) the victory of God & my Saviour. Therefore a glorious light shone in my head. My soul was cast into the hand of my dear Saviour by faith. As Mr. H. took me by the hand crossing the pure water, I felt a thrill of crying for joy, though not one drop of a tear fell in sight from my eyes. I acknowledged the hand of my God was laid upon my trembling soul, also how merciful & loving he was within me. I did not have any fear nor trouble in the least, because my trust & hope were in my Redeemer. My dear father & a gentleman aided me up out of the water, & I sat in the chair with the wet clothes, on utterance of another prayer. I went to church & the holy communion. Mr. H. gave me the right hand of fellowship in God. It was a most glorious & pious Sunday, ever more for me to retain (remember). I have written this for you, my dear friends, Eliza & Elvira Rogers.

After the death of her father and the consequent breaking up of the family, she had some anxious thoughts about her future support, but was relieved by an arrangement which Dr. Howe made, whereby a home in the Institution was secured to her. On my return to this country, after an absence of two years and a half, she wrote me the following letter, expressing her gratitude : —

HANOVER, Nov. 26, 1871.
MY DEAR FRIEND MRS. LAMSON :
I had a long letter from Miss R. two weeks since, & was highly delighted to hear about your return. I have

planned for departing for Lebanon next Saturday, to
visit my sisters. I rejoice in the mercy of God for
his kind providence, that a home at the Inst. is designed for my abode as long as I would like. Mother
had a cordial & welcome letter from Dr. H. last winter.
I shall be entirely welcome to the Institution, & devolve
upon their kind care & so it is no pay for my board, but
it is an expressive (?) home for me since my dear father
is above the heavens. Next Tuesday is three years of
his death in peace of our Savior, so he has been in a
glorious world three years long. My home here is
broken up. I cannot enjoy this life so much. I wish
much to see you & talk constantly with you. Do be
prompt to call on my birthday 21st of December or
sooner. I long to see you at Inst. I dread the cold
climate of N. H. Give my best regards to Mr. L. &
love to the dear ones. God bless you. Believe me
your ever loving friend,

LAURA.

Until 1876 she had lost by death no one who
had ever stood in the relation of teacher to her,
and I doubt if she had ever thought that any of
us might die before herself. Dr. Howe had for
months been in failing health, and she had seen
but little of him for a year. He had been absent
from Boston much of the time, and when at home
was too weak to bear the excitement of talking
with her. She was told that he was very ill and
that it was feared he could not live. A few hours
before his death it was thought that it might be a

comfort to her to visit him, and she was led beside the bed on which he lay unconscious. Very gently she passed her hand over his face; her tears flowed freely, but she did not allow herself to make a sound. She realized fully the loss she was to sustain. For many years of her early life in Boston she had been a member of his private family, and had felt as if she were his child, and when in later years her home was with the blind, she had daily expected his kind greeting and words of cheer, and now, as she took leave of him, she knew that she had lost her best earthly friend and greatest benefactor.

A few days after she wrote to me as follows: —

S. BOSTON, Jan. 30, '76.

MY DEAR FRIEND:

I am sitting in the love of our heavenly Father who is ever good to bless us with his sun to-day. I am in my sunny cosy room this A. M. Your letter came to me with much welcome & joy. There is a good deal (of) comfort in much sunshine, though it tries my feelings in thought of never meeting & grasping my best & noble friend Dr. Howe on earth. The path seems so desolate & void without sight of him to us all. But Jesus is all & in all. He fills our way with light & sunshine. I think much of Dr. H. day & night, with sorrow, & gratitude, & love, & sincerity. . . .

Her health was seriously affected by her sorrow, and when she left us the following summer to go to her mother, it seemed doubtful if she lived to return.

Another sorrow followed closely, in the loss of her beloved friend and teacher, Miss Rogers. With characteristic thoughtfulness of others, she requested me, on my last visit to her, to write Laura of her extreme illness, and thus prevent the shock of the sudden announcement of her death. In my letter, which was accidentally delayed a fortnight on its way, I suggested to Laura that she should send a last message to her dear friend. She wrote at once the following letter, which was only received by her friend a few days before her decease : —

HANOVER, June 25, 1876.

MY VERY DEAR MISS ROGERS:

I received a letter from Mrs. Lamson yesterday, but it was forgotten since its arrival, several weeks ago. I was at Lebanon visiting my dear sisters for more than two weeks then. I am very sorrowful for your dear sisters and parents, who feel so grievously afflicted with the idea of missing you at the gracious calling of the loving Father. You shall receive a crown of eternal life from heaven. You will have a holy home forever. Your sisters & parents will be comforted by the God of comfort. God is very gentle in all his dealings with those who love & hope & trust him.

We shall all meet in a glorious world where there is no sorrow nor pain nor parting. I joy of meeting Dr. Howe & my dear father & friends. My mother & I join in ardent love & sympathy to you & the family. I should like to have a little token from you, for its sake in remembrance of my dearly loved friend & teacher

Truly your loving friend,

L. D. BRIDGMAN.

To a sister of Miss Rogers she wrote the following letter: —

S. BOSTON, April 22, 1877.

MY DEAR FRIEND ELVIRA:

It is a rainy & languid morning. I thank you truly for a nice letter which you wrote to me last summer. You must come to see me shortly, as I anticipate to leave here first week of June, & go to Troy, N. H., to visit the wife of my parents' old & excellent minister for some weeks. I ought to have replied to your welcome letter long, long ago, but have been so procrastinate, & also so ambitiously busy, & had many ill spells too. I do not enjoy strong health as I am growing old. I long to fly to my everlasting home with God. It is life's weary journey for me to bear until death take place. You & I shall be happy to meet dear Miss Rogers in a holy home which is heaven. . . . I presume, of course, that you call on your poor & lonely parents very frequently. Who is with them in the absence of their dear daughter, E. R.? I realize how hard it is for them to miss her during their old age. But it is short ere they will go to the glorious world above. You may like to dwell in their house & keep house for your own, & console the old people with your society. Please to remember me kindly to Mr. G. & your relatives. I should be so happy to call on you & friends in Billerica. Let me hear from you as soon as you get my letter. I feel so tired continually beyond my strength. I was sickly last spring until in Aug. I was much more like my own self, although it seems as if I might not live many years, I feel so frail God cares for me & I trust in his loving providence & in his tender mercy. I shall be hoping to see you soon. I miss Dr. Howe so sadly & loved him as a father.

Truly your loving friend,

LAURA BRIDGMAN.

One more incident showing her kindness of heart deserves mention. She was invited to visit some friends, and on arriving at their house, found them away from home. On their return, they explained what had seemed to her discourteous, saying they had been to visit a little boy, the son of a clergyman, who had lately met with a sad accident; while jumping on a car he had had both feet taken off. Her sympathies were so much excited that she could think of little else. On returning home she interested the blind pupils, and a contribution of ten dollars was sent by them to the little sufferer, to assist in the purchase of artificial feet. She wrote to him a note of sympathy.

JAN. 2, 1877.

DEAR LITTLE FELLOW,

Whom I pity most sorrowfully. God is gentle in his dealings towards them who are sorely afflicted. Casting your care on God for he cares for you. Be of good cheer. I hope that you may be blessed with a kind providence as long as you live. God will make your life his care. You will promote much happiness of others by the Holy Spirit. You will be a devout disciple of our blest Savior. He will redeem you from evil & cleanse you with His precious blood. I heard of you with grief & sympathy, last evening. I came to visit Mr. & Mrs. Heywood yesterday. I wish you many happy new Years.

LAURA D. BRIDGMAN.

CHAPTER XX.

In a life so quiet as that of Laura has been for the last eight years, there is little to furnish further material for the journalist. She spends the summer and early autumn with her relatives and friends in New Hampshire, and for the remainder of the year her home is at the Institution, in one of the four cottages which are occupied by the blind girls. Here she is under the kind care of Miss Wood, and enjoys making herself useful by assisting in some light work about the house. Her room has a window towards the south, and she often dates her letters "Sunny Home," showing her appreciation of the blessing of sunshine. She takes pleasure in decorating it with the little things which have been given her, and in asking her intimate friends to make their visits there, so that she can display them.

Her habits of industry which were formed in childhood are a blessing to her now, and she never finds time hang heavily upon her hands.

Through the kindness of friends she has received gifts of books and magazines printed in raised type at the different presses of the country, and these, with the Bible and Memoir of Dr. Howe, form her little library, and are a source of great enjoyment to her. She has made many friends, chiefly ladies who have been so much interested in her as to learn to converse in the manual alphabet. Occasional calls from them and an extensive correspondence add much to her pleasure. She sews, knits, crochets lace, mats, and other fancy articles, which she sells to visitors with her autograph attached, thereby increasing her income.

Her appearance is that of a very delicate person, and she impresses all who see her by her apparent frailness, though for the last year she has been in better health than for some time previous. The regular life she leads, with its freedom from care and anxiety and excitement, has given her strength to overcome sickness which threatened to be serious. She has never been a sound sleeper.

Some of her expressions previously quoted may lead the reader to think that she is inclined to despondency, and thus convey a false impression of her mental condition.

It is true that she has, even from the days of her childhood, enjoyed telling of her illnesses, and receiving the sympathy of her friends, but with so few subjects for thought as she has in comparison with others, it would be remarkable if her own feelings did not form the first topic of conversation. She turns afterward to other subjects of mutual interest, enjoys a joke, and appreciates a witty remark.

She speaks sometimes of the long walks we used to take, and the thought that she has not equal strength now causes her to utter a sound indicating regret, but she does not seem to dwell upon it, or to be made unhappy by it for any length of time.

The remainder of her life will be shadowed by her late bereavement, but we have seen in her letters the light of her earnest faith shining through the darkness.

Those who have constant intercourse with her bear testimony to the great change that has taken place in her character. She never manifests anger now and is always kind and gentle. In speaking with me lately of her former experience and of the frequency with which she gave way to passion, she said, "Sometimes I feel tempted to anger, but I can resist it now. God gives me strength."

She has written, within a few years, two compositions which she calls "poems." The first is on "Light and Darkness." As she has access to very little poetry in the books she can read herself, and she seems not to have aimed at any imitation of this, we think she must have taken the general idea from some parts of the Bible.

Light represents day.
Light is more brilliant than ruby, even **diamond.**
Light is whiter than snow.
Darkness is night like.
It looks as black as iron.
Darkness is a sorrow.
Joy is a thrilling rapture.
Light yields a shooting joy through the human (heart)
Light is sweet as honey, but
Darkness is bitter as salt, and more than vinegar.
Light is finer than gold and even finest gold.
Joy is a real light.
Joy is a blazing flame.
Darkness is frosty.
A good sleep is a white curtain,
A bad sleep is a black curtain.

In bringing these notes to a close, let me express the hope that they will be the means of gaining for Laura many appreciative friends. Few lives of men or women could bear the test of such scrutiny as hers has received, which indeed would not have been justifiable for the satisfaction of curiosity, but only for its value to the scholar.

In her declining years she will be tenderly cared for by those to whose trust she was committed by him who was so many years her friend and protector; and when the arm of an earthly friend can no longer be her support and guide, and she walks " through the valley of the shadow of death," may she " fear no evil," but rest on the arm of Him

Holy home.

Heaven is holy home

Holy home is from ever.

lasting to everlasting.

Holy home is summery.

I pass this dark home

toward a Light home.

Earthly home shall perish.

But holy home shall end.

ure for ever,

Earthly home is Wintery.

Hard it is for us to apprec

iate the radiance of holy

home because of blind,
ness of our minds.
How glorious holy home
is, a still more than a
beam of sun.
By the finger of God
my eyes & ears shall
be opened.
The string of my tongue
shall be loosed.
With sweeter joys in
Heaven of shall heart.e
speak & see.

With glorious rapture in
holy home for me to bear
the Angels sing & perform
up on Instruments.
    Also that I can behold
the beauty of Heavenly
                home.
Jesus Christ has gone
to prepare a place for
those who Love & believe
him.
My zealous hope is that
sinners might turn them

selves from the power
of darkness unto light
divine.
When I die. God will
make me happy.
In Heaven music is
sweeter than honey, a
finer than a diamond.
L. D. Bridgman.

whom she sincerely loves and who has promised to be her leader to the heavenly home of which she writes in the following poem : —

HOLY HOME.

Heaven is holy home.
Holy home is from everlasting to everlasting.
Holy home is summerly.
I pass this dark home toward a light home.
Earthly home shall perish,
But holy home shall endure forever.
Earthly home is wintery.
Hard it is for us to appreciate the radiance of holy
    home because of blindness of our minds.
How glorious holy home is, and still more than a beam
    of sun !
By the finger of God my eyes and ears shall be opened.
The string of my tongue shall be loosed.
With sweeter joys in heaven I shall hear and speak and
    see.
With glorious rapture in holy home for me to hear the
    Angels sing and perform upon instruments.
Also that I can behold the beauty of Heavenly home.
Jesus Christ has gone to prepare a place for those who
    love and believe him.
My zealous hope is that sinners might turn themselves
    from the power of darkness unto light divine.
When I die, God will make me happy.
In Heaven music is sweeter than honey, and finer than
    a diamond.

L. D. BRIDGMAN.

APPENDIX.

OLIVER CASWELL'S FIRST LESSON.

FOR the benefit of any future case of similar affliction, I have thought it desirable to describe minutely
the first lesson given to Oliver Caswell, a deaf, dumb,
and blind boy who entered the Institution at South
Boston, Sept. 30, 1841, at the age of twelve years, having lost his senses when three years and four months
old by scarlet fever.   Lucy Reed, also deaf, dumb, and
blind, had been received in the previous February, but
remained only five months, having returned to her
home two months previous to Oliver's arrival.

Not having become acquainted with Laura until she
had been two years and a half under instruction, I was
much interested in watching Lucy's progress, the
course of training being the same as that which was
adopted for Laura, and which has been described in
the preceding pages.   Four months elapsed before
Lucy attached any significance to the process she was
required to go through several times a day, of feeling
the letters in raised type composing the various labels,
which were placed upon a few common objects, and
moving her fingers in certain directions to correspond
with them.   Her ungoverned will and stolid indifference were undoubtedly serious obstacles to her progress,
but it had taken more than two months before Laura

24

received the idea, although she was a most interested scholar. After a careful study of our work with Lucy, it seemed to me that the introduction of the raised letters at the beginning of the training was entirely useless, and resulted only in a serious complication of the whole matter. No one would teach a little child to read until it had learned to talk, so the deaf and blind child should only be taught to spell the names of objects on the fingers, and not to read the raised letters at the same time; the attention being thus concentrated on this one point, I believe the desired result would be far more speedily attained

I had often expressed the wish that one more such child might be brought to us, that my theory might be tested, and on this Sept. 30th I was made happy by a summons from Dr. Howe, and the announcement that such a child had arrived, and I might begin my experiment at once, while he was absent in the city.

That there need be nothing to distract attention, I led the boy into a room where we could be undisturbed, and seated myself beside him upon a sofa. He first wished to find what manner of person I was, and I gave him all the opportunity he desired to examine the arrangement of my hair, to feel of my face, dress, chain, breastpin, rings, etc., until his curiosity was satisfied. Next he examined the sofa on which we were seated, and then rested quietly. Now was my time to attract his attention. I led him to a door, and placed his hand upon the key which was in the lock. He made the motion of turning it, nodding with a quizzical look, all which meant plainly, Yes, I know what a key is for, did you suppose I did not? Taking the key from the door, we returned to the sofa. Now he was curious to know what was to come next. I placed his hand upon the key, then lifting it, moved the fingers in the positions for the letters k-e-y, repeating it several times. Then I placed my hand in his and let him feel that I moved my fingers in the same way. By tapping his hand he understood that he was to repeat it himself; he succeeded in making k, but needed assistance on the other letters, which was given by letting him feel me make them again. On the second trial he spelled the word without assistance. The expression on his face now indicated, I wonder what all this means. Next I took a mug from a table near by, and placed it in his hand. Again he nodded and raised it to his lips, tipping it as a sign of drinking. Laying his hand upon it, as I had done before with the key, I moved his fingers to make the letters m-u-g, repeating it with my own fingers, his hand resting on mine so that he could feel the motions, and then asked him by a sign to do it himself. After three efforts he was successful, and showed pleasure in receiving a pat upon his head as a sign of approbation. Then I returned to the key. He had forgotten those letters, but after feeling me make them once, succeeded in spelling it. Turning back to the mug, he remembered two letters, and after a few trials more, spelled each correctly without assistance. All this time his face wore a puzzled look mingled with indifference, which would perhaps have triumphed at this point but for his spirit of obedience, which prompted him to do as he perceived I wished. These two words learned, he sat back upon the sofa as if to say, This is enough of such nonsense. Just then I drew a pin from my dress and handed it to him. He made the sign of sticking it into his coat, and listlessly returned it to me. I lifted his hand, which he had lain quietly on his knee, and spelled with my fingers p-i-n. With a nervous movement and an expression of face quite unlike anything he had exhibited before, he tapped my hand, showing his wish that I should repeat it, and then, without waiting to make the letters himself, with a look of intense earnestness, he sprung from the sofa and drew me to the table, placing his hands upon it, and then rapping my fingers. As I made the letters t-a-b-l-e, he perceived that they were unlike those he had learned for the key, mug, and pin. His countenance became radiant. He led me rapidly about the room, putting my hands on different objects, and feeling me spell the names. A half-hour had passed since we took the key from the door, and he had received the idea which it had taken four months to give to Lucy Reed and nearly three months to Laura. The success of the experiment was far beyond my expectations. Had we saved a month's time it would have been a great gain ; but the work was done, when I supposed it only commenced. Once having received the idea that objects have names, and that by movements of our fingers we can communicate them, the remaining work is simply to acquire a knowledge of those movements. In teaching a deaf, dumb, and blind person, the Frenchman's maxim is eminently true, " C'est le premier pas qui coute."

It will be noticed that in selecting the words to be taught, care was taken that they should be as short as possible, and that no letter used in the name of one object should be repeated in that of another. This is very important, as the first idea which the mind receives is probably the difference in the words, and by making any part of them similar we make this less striking.

Let no one who undertakes a similar work be discouraged, if, in following the steps above described, it takes weeks or even months to attain the desired result. but in no case can the labels be of assistance.

CPSIA information can be obtained at www.ICGtesting.com
Printed in the USA
VOW100747220312

253LV00004B/71/P